Religion, Flesh, and Blood

Religion, Flesh, and Blood

The Convergence of HIV/AIDS, Black Sexual Expression, and Therapeutic Religion

Pamela Leong

LEXINGTON BOOKS
Lanham • Boulder • New York • London

Published by Lexington Books
An imprint of The Rowman & Littlefield Publishing Group, Inc.
4501 Forbes Boulevard, Suite 200, Lanham, Maryland 20706
www.rowman.com

Unit A, Whitacre Mews, 26-34 Stannary Street, London SE11 4AB

British Library Cataloguing in Publication Information Available

Library of Congress Cataloging-in-Publication Data

Leong, Pamela.
Religion, flesh, and blood : the convergence of HIV/AIDS, black sexual expression, and therapeutic
religion / Pamela Leong.
pages cm.
Includes bibliographical references and index.
ISBN 978-0-7391-9442-3 (cloth : alk. paper) — ISBN 978-0-7391-9443-0 (electronic)
) 1. Medicine—Religious aspects—Christianity—Case studies. 2. Unity Fellowship of Christ
Church, Los Angeles. 3. HIV infections—Religious aspects—Christianity. 4. AIDS (Disease)—
Religious aspects—Christianity. 5. African Americans—Religion. I. Title.
BT732.2.L46 2015
289.9—dc23

2015004339

∞ ™ The paper used in this publication meets the minimum requirements of American
National Standard for Information Sciences Permanence of Paper for Printed Library
Materials, ANSI/NISO Z39.48-1992.

Printed in the United States of America

Contents

Acknowledgments

A number of people have helped me craft this book, and others have supported me in countless other ways. However, I will not include a rolling list of everyone I know here, or everyone I have met in my entire life. Nor do I wish to name drop high-profile people who may have inspired me but with whom I have no direct relationship whatsoever and may have never even met. Instead, I wish to acknowledge the people who have helped me craft this book in substantive ways, and those who have supported me in the process consistently and unfailingly.

First, I thank all the people who have mentored me academically and who have provided valuable feedback about drafts of the project in which this book is based. Foremost, I am indebted to Paul Lichterman and Donald E. Miller, my dissertation committee co-chairs at the University of Southern California.

I thank the people and organizations who have assisted me financially while I was in the depths of the data collection and data analysis process, and also in the depths of impoverishment as a graduate school student. The Department of Sociology at the University of Southern California provided full support and funding throughout all of my graduate school years. The Center of Religion and Civic Culture at USC provided a dissertation grant that allowed me to fund the bulk of my research. I also thank Ms. Wallis Annenberg for the Wallis Annenberg Fellowship, which allowed me to work full-time on the project in 2004–2005 without competing responsibilities. My mother, Barbara Leong, provided some financial help during my graduate school years--both large and small--for which I am extremely grateful.

My deepest gratitude to my publisher, Lexington Books/Rowman & Littlefield. Special thanks especially to the following individuals: editors Joseph Parry and Jana Hodges-Kluck; assistant editor Sarah Craig; and assistant production editor Macrae Stone. There likely were many other nameless individuals who helped produce this book, and I thank them too.

Throughout the intensive research process (graduate school and onward), my mother steadfastly remained a source of motivation, inspiration, support, humor, and love, even during days, months, and years that felt darkest, loneliest, and bleakest.

Lastly, I am indebted to the Archbishop Carl Bean and the men and women of Unity Fellowship Church and the Minority AIDS Project. The church, the outreach organization, and the people who represent the two communities are what motivated this research project in the first place. It was a very long journey, but one that was full of joy, tears, humor, and, always, love and compassion. Thank you, Archbishop Bean, for your vision and for your humanity.

Chapter One

The Therapeutic Ethic

HIV/AIDS: THE LOOMING CLOUD IN BLACK RELIGIOUS AMERICA

Jackie, a petite, sixty-four-year-old, African-American woman, worked as a bartender at a bar and nightclub frequented by gay African-American men and women when the AIDS epidemic hit the United States. The epidemic proved devastating, killing many of Jackie's friends, acquaintances, and customers. As she described it, "[W]hen [the AIDS epidemic] hit, it went through the bar like this. I mean five, six, seven, eight [deaths]. . . . You have a funeral at 9:00 in the morning. One at 12:00. And a panic hit the gay, black community." Back then, nobody knew what AIDS was, and the general public believed that people could contract AIDS simply through casual contact. Initially, the epidemic appeared to be confined to the homosexual population. But "then it hit the church circle, and that's when folks started to get scared. They don't care about the folks in the bar."

Jackie had a friend who was a life-long member and servant of a Church of God and Christ (COGIC). This friend had worked in the COGIC bookstore. When he died of AIDS, "They would not allow his body to come in the church. We had to get together and have his service at the funeral service, and they sent two people to speak up. And he worked every day in their bookstore!" This account suggests that even life-long servants of certain denominations or congregations are not guaranteed congregational loyalty in return, if one is exposed as gay or, even worse, a gay individual stricken with AIDS. In the case of Jackie's friend, in spite of his dedication and commitment to his church, when his time case, the church let him down. "And that's what was happening with a lot of the churches," Jackie pointed out. ". . . And it still is."

1

Candy, a forty-five-year-old, African-American, post-operative male-to-female transgender, added that her mother mentioned that the choir director who had served at a church in Chicago "for years and years" passed away (presumably from HIV/AIDS) and the church would not hold the funeral services at the church. Instead, the funeral services were held at a mortuary. Candy asserted, "Wow! That is unbelievable. That is truly unbelievable. In this day and time . . . that kind of stuff is still happening. But that just shows where we haven't reached out to enough places yet." She wondered, "Can you imagine going to a church all your life and paying your tithes and die, and then they won't give you a funeral?"

Jones, a forty-year-old, light-skinned, biracial male, elaborated that African-American churches are "still trapped in the idea that AIDS is God's punishment on gay people. They got twenty years' [worth of] thinking going on. 'Cause they believe what some white man told them. And they went right along with it, instead of asking questions, disseminating information [to the effect of], 'Oh, it's a gay people's thing. Well, I ain't gay. I ain't gotta worry about it.'" Rodney, a fifty-year-old, HIV-positive, African American, gay male, concurred. "A lot of them [black churches] still think [AIDS] is a gay, white disease." In fact, as a consultant at a community-based AIDS organization, clients would approach Rodney and proclaim that "Black people don't get AIDS." He explained, "It's a denial thing, but I don't know how you can be in denial when you see the numbers and the rate of infections."

The numbers are all too telling. African Americans comprise about 13 percent of the U.S. population,[1] and yet they are grossly over-represented in terms of the rates of HIV/AIDS. Since the beginning of the AIDS epidemic, African Americans have accounted for 40 percent of the total AIDS cases diagnosed. One half of the estimated new numbers of HIV/AIDS diagnoses in the United States in 2004 were for African Americans.[2] The rate shrank slightly to 44 percent in 2010, but considering the smaller size of the African-American population, the 2010 HIV infection rate is staggering, representing a rate that is eight times the rate of new HIV infections among whites.[3]

By the end of 2010, over 260,000 African Americans diagnosed with AIDS will have died and new HIV cases among African Americans are anticipated. The Centers for Disease Control and Prevention estimate that 1 in 16 African-American men and 1 in 32 African-American women will become HIV-positive at some point in their lifetime.[4] Once infected, African Americans have shorter survival times, and experience more deaths from HIV/AIDS than any other racial group. In 2010 alone, African Americans represented nearly 50 percent of all HIV deaths,[5] with African-American men seven times more likely than white men to die from HIV/AIDS, and African-American women 15 times more likely than white women to die from the disease.[6]

The statistics confirm just how profound the racial disparities are with respect to HIV/AIDS. From the onset of disease and continuing through the HIV continuum of care and, inevitably, death, African Americans face worse outcomes. Unfortunately, salt is added to the wounds of African Americans who are GLBT and/or HIV-positive or HIV-at-risk when deeply important social institutions in the black community alienate them.

BALANCING A FINE LINE: EXPLAINING AFRICAN-AMERICAN CONGREGATIONAL RETICENCE TO RESPOND TO HIV/AIDS

History has demonstrated that African-American churches are very progressive with respect to a number of social issues. It is curious, then, that these churches have been relatively reticent to become involved in HIV/AIDS-related efforts, even in light of the disproportionate rates of HIV/AIDS infection among African Americans. This highlights a contradiction among black churches:[7] While they are perceived to be important instruments for liberating African Americans from oppression, they simultaneously represent what is likely one of the most conservative institutions within African-American communities. Such a contradiction seems to pull black worshippers in two directions.

AIDS activists have questioned whether African-American religious institutions and clergy are following Christian tenets when they avert the AIDS issue. Activists have argued that Christianity mandates that Christ take care of the sick, but that the churches have acted "un-Christ-like" by failing to care for the people most affected by HIV/AIDS—intravenous drug users and gays and lesbians, with the latter particularly neglected.[8] These critiques highlight the divisive nature of HIV/AIDS among African-American congregations. On the one hand, African-American churches have traditionally provided services and care to those in need, regardless of their social status. On the other hand, conservative Christian ideals command that these same churches distance themselves from "immoral" individuals (e.g., drug addicts, gays, and HIV-positive men and women).

One line of argument claims that the black religious community's silence with respect to HIV/AIDS stems from a reluctance to discuss issues of sexuality and, in particular, homosexuality, a situation compounded by many African Americans' continuing perception of AIDS as an exclusively "gay" disease. Although such attitudes have abated over time, some black religious leaders continue to frame HIV/AIDS as a "moral problem," in which case HIV/AIDS-affected individuals are perceived in binary terms: Those who contract HIV through blood transfusions or through maternal transmission are deemed to be "innocent" victims and are therefore deserving of our sympathy, while those who contract HIV sexually or through intravenous drug use are thought to be undeserving of our sympathies and protection, given the onset-controllability of the disease. But in distancing themselves from what they view are HIV-prone gay individuals in particular, black religious leaders conveniently dissociate themselves from what they deem are the less desirable members of their own community and engage in what Cathy Cohen terms "secondary marginalization,"[9] impeding efforts to curb HIV/AIDS in black communities.

Reginald Glenn Blaxton even maintains that the black church is more conservative than its white evangelical Protestant counterpart and that African Americans, in general, tend to be more conservative than white Americans on a range of social issues other than issues of racial justice.[10] Weatherford and Weatherford[11] note the tendency for African Americans to take the Bible literally, particularly with respect to sexual matters.

However, it is too simplistic to state that black churches are necessarily more homophobic or conservative in religious doctrine than other churches with respect to HIV/AIDS. The situation for black churches is far more complex. First, homophobia and HIV/AIDS represent two additional strikes against a population that already faces multiple strikes by larger American society. After generations of being sexually violated, as well as sexually stereotyped, it is difficult for African Americans to discuss sexuality of any type, and not just homosexuality. Charges of black hypersexuality have long been common,[12] which may hint to an underlying reason why African-American religious leaders have avoided matters involving sexuality. Second, HIV/AIDS evokes not only questions about sexual attitudes and behaviors, but moral meanings of sickness, plague, and death. In this way, HIV/AIDS evokes multiple emotions that range from guilt and shame to unsettling fear.[13]

Black churches' silence with respect to HIV/AIDS is further complicated by theories that associate African-Americans' disproportionate contraction of HIV with genocide. The conspiracy and genocide theories take various perspectives. A 1990 study found more than one third of the 1,000 African-American church members surveyed in five cities believed that the AIDS virus was deliberately created in a germ warfare laboratory in order to eliminate blacks.[14] Other perspectives maintain that the U.S. government's gross disregard of crises that occur in African-American communities—which include joblessness, poverty, drug addiction, and AIDS—is indicative of genocidal intent on the part of the U.S. government. Still, another perspective views the U.S. government as purposefully engaged in practices detrimental to the welfare and well-being of African Americans, including the promotion of drug addiction and overdoses, violence, and HIV contraction,[15] in order to eradicate African-American individuals and communities.

The most cited evidence of African-American genocide, however, is the Tuskegee Syphilis Study, which has now become the symbol of scientific/ medical racism. Between 1932 and 1972, the Public Health Service (now the Centers for Disease Control) conducted research on 600 African-American men, 399 of whom had syphilis, and deliberately withheld treatment from the syphilis-infected men in order to study the progression of the disease. The participants were not informed that they had the disease, were prevented from receiving care, and their sexual partners were not provided precautions. It is estimated that around 28 to 100 African-American men died from complications of syphilis.[16]

HIV/AIDS emerged only a decade or so after the Tuskegee experiment, fueling genocidal beliefs among some African Americans, particularly in light of the incurable nature of the disease and the inevitable fatality associated with AIDS. With this historical context, perhaps it is understandable that African-American clergy have been silent on the AIDS issue, because it inevitably evokes past governmental exploitation, mistreatment, and intentional neglect of African Americans. In this way, silence by African-American clergy speaks volumes, alluding to the damage to the black American psyche as a result of prior exploitation, and the ensuing distrust of medical and governmental interventions in African-American affairs.

To complicate matters, given the perceived onset-controllability of HIV, larger society may believe that African Americans have only themselves to blame for their disproportionate rates of HIV/AIDS. The debate over the origin of HIV/AIDS in Africa or Haiti[17] likely also intensified the condemnation of African Americans, displacing the blame for the entire AIDS epidemic onto those of African origin. HIV/AIDS and all of its implications, then, would only serve to further malign the reputation of African Americans.

For all of these reasons, there is considerable pressure on black churches and black religious leaders to function as the representatives and moral centers of black communities. As representatives of moral authority, black religious leaders and churches may feel obligated to present themselves as morally pure, particularly since they are acutely aware that larger society tends to perceive African Americans in pathological terms.[18] Openly tolerating homosexuality and bisexuality, thus, especially in the more biblically-oriented churches, may mark black churches as contaminated or deviant, but the contamination may extend beyond the neighborhood or community context to society at large, implicating the African-American population collectively. Because black churches represent one of the few institutions respected by the white majority, black religious leaders and community members are cautious to avoid anything that could mar the reputation and integrity of their churches.[19, 20] Potentially maligning positions include a public tolerance, or even simply acknowledgment, of homosexuality, bisexuality, and/or illicit substance use.

Hence, the reticence by African-American religious leaders to address the AIDS problem may be less attributable to their denial of the severity of HIV/AIDS in African-American communities, or to their denial of HIV-risk behaviors, and more imputable to their rejection of racist assumptions about African-American sexuality and behaviors and the ensuing efforts by whites to socially control African Americans. Unfortunately, this silence and denial come at a great cost to the well-being, health, and survival of African Americans.

UNDERSCORING THE IMPORTANCE OF BLACK CONGREGATIONS

The importance of religion and the church for African Americans has been well documented. From the start, black religion has played a pivotal role in the survival and rebellion of African slaves, and it continues to be a central catalyst of change for African Americans in contemporary times. A broad range of literatures—ranging from the works of Myrdal[21] and Mays and Nicholson[22] to more contemporary scholars such as Morris[23] and Lincoln and Mamiya[24]—documents the many ways in which black religion and black religious institutions have been instrumental in the development of black communities, promoting both the individual and collective well-being of African Americans.

Historically, the black church functioned as more than a place of worship. Foremost, it represents political independence for African-American people: It is a symbolic extension of the freedom and independence of all African-American people.[25] Specifically, because the black church, for the most part, is autonomous, relatively immune from external surveillance by the white majority,[26] and there is greater freedom from white interference and violence, the decision-making of the religious body therefore rests entirely in the hands of African Americans themselves.[27]

Second, the church represents an economic power base for African Americans, because it is one of the few institutions that African Americans independently own, operate, and control in a society shaped by a political-economic ideology and structure that disproportionately obstructs wealth attainment by racial/ethnic minorities and the poor.[28] Third, the black church symbolizes a revolutionary instrument: It represents a major site for meeting, political organization, and contestation by African Americans, and it is a vehicle for raising black consciousness. The ability for black religious leaders to raise consciousness increases the potential for collective social action and social change by African Americans.

African-American churches and religious leaders consistently have responded to various forms of oppression—notably chronic legal discrimination and racial prejudice—through innovative means, after which other marginalized populations themselves have modeled. African-American churches also have improved the social status of African Americans through the advocacy for better economic opportunities, housing, and schooling. The churches have nurtured and encouraged the self-respect of their parishioners, and have used spiritual resources to support black pride and achievements.[29]

Black religious institutions are important in other ways. In urban communities, where racial minorities and the poor tend to be concentrated, and where, not coincidentally, poverty and its pathological by-products, including HIV/AIDS, are prevalent, churches have long played a key role as refuges from oppression, spaces for social mobilization, cultural centers, leadership development institutes, providers of social services and support, agents of socialization and acculturation, educational institutes, and pulpits for visionaries. In fact, in many devastated neighborhoods, churches are among the oldest and most established community institutions, and they are well-received because they are committed to combating the "ideology of despair, materialism, and cynicism" that pervades these low-income urban communities.[30] Religious institutions, in fact, have credibility and roots in urban low-income communities, and clergy are considered respected, credible, and trustworthy sources of information and guidance, a crucial point for low-income and ethnic minority individuals and groups, who tend to be more distrusting of public officials and public agency workers.[31]

Thus, without the support of their religious institutions, traditionally a backbone in African-American communities, African Americans with low socioeconomic status who identify as GLBT and/or who are HIV-positive or HIV-at-risk may feel even more displaced from the social world. This radical separation from the social world is what Peter Berger terms "anomy."[32] Anomy, and the ensuing feeling of hopelessness, is a powerful threat to the individual, because it severs satisfying social ties, inflicts psychological tensions, and potentially produces a sense of meaninglessness for individuals for whom religion and spirituality play pivotal roles.

Despite the prominence of the church in African-American communities, a few contemporary religion scholars have cautioned against broadly painting the black church as the bastion for social change for African Americans. Omar McRoberts, for instance, maintains that rather than assuming that black churches are automatic and direct participants in efforts toward political, social, and economic change, the ecological context must be considered. Specifically, the church's relationship in the neighborhood—its level of attachment to the surrounding area—shape the church's level of grass-roots activism. In *Streets of Glory*, his study of storefront churches in low-income, black urban neighborhoods in the Boston area, McRoberts discovered that it was people who lived outside of the neighborhoods who were active in the churches; they actively participated, supported, and ran the churches in large part because of the low overhead costs (e.g., low rents). But because the church members were not neighborhood residents, they had little attachment to the neighborhood and therefore were less likely to engage in grass-roots efforts for the betterment of the neighborhood. Thus, rather than serving as neighborhood niche churches that focused on the interests and needs of the community members in the immediate vicinity, the storefront churches carved out particular niches for very specific target populations.[33]

Marla Frederick's research also, in some ways, knocks down the idea of the black church as the singular vanguard institution for social change in matters that affect African-American communities. In her ethnography of a Baptist church community in Halifax County, North Carolina, Frederick de-emphasizes the institutional factors of the black church—its structures and cultural practices—and instead gives weight to the personal forms of spirituality of church-going women. The implication is that it is the personal spirituality, rather than the institutional influences, that sustains and inspires the church-going women to engage in community service, even in the face of socioeconomic disenfranchisement.[34] Hence, it is not an abstract entity—"the black church"—that is given the sole credit as the agent of social change; rather, the individual church-going women themselves are recognized as engaged beings and social activists.

THE PURPOSE OF THIS STUDY

While critiques of the mystification of the black church are certainly warranted, there is no denial that the church remains a prominent part of the culture and survival of African Americans. Moreover, in spite of the constraints and pressures that black churches face, and the continuing homophobic environment that characterizes some of the more mainstream churches, black congregations remain crucial in the fight against HIV/AIDS in African-American communities, and in the survival of African-American GLBT and HIV-affected worshippers. Currently, there is an absence of ethnographic and other qualitative works that focus on African-American AIDS ministries, let alone any AIDS ministries. This study aims to fill that gap. Specifically, this study strives to provide insight as to why one African-American congregation is able to: 1) transcend constraints imposed by traditional religious institutions; 2) address the health, spiritual, and social needs of its parishioners without losing sight of its religious traditions; and 3) at all times, maintain an AIDS-activist orientation.

Although the case study focuses on an AIDS ministry, this book is not about the delivery of physical health care. Rather, the book is oriented toward the cultural components of a religious organization, and how these elements help temper the shame, fear, and other distress associated with marginalized social statuses. Focusing on the religious and cultural strategies rather than on programmatic efforts or medical health care services for those stricken by HIV/AIDS, I argue that the congregation's distinct therapeutic culture enables members to reconcile religious contradictions.

This book focuses on the processes involved in creating and maintaining a religious environment that affirms the stigmatized statuses of its members, with an eye to understanding how the congregation is able to reconcile religious contradictions. The study highlights the role of religious culture. Specifically, the focus is on the language of a religious faith that is therapeutically oriented, allowing for a reconciliation of religious contradictions. By underscoring the importance of religious language and patterns of communication, and how these shape congregational rituals, practices, and social action, the purpose of this study is to examine the distinct ways in which religion is articulated in order to legitimize and affirm social differences, and to promote the interests and well-being of marginalized individuals and groups.

THE THERAPEUTIC ETHIC AND THERAPEUTIC RELIGION

The therapeutic ethic is a tradition of individualism that centers around self-discovery, uniqueness, autonomy, personal experiences, self-expressions, open communication, personal growth, and self-fulfillment.[35, 36, 37, 38, 39] This book focuses on one religious community that blends therapy and religion, producing a "therapeutic religion"[40] in which: the role, meaning, and meaningfulness of religion are open to interpretation; religious identities are shaped by life experiences; healing of the religious person is underscored; and the highly personalized forms of religion, although individualized, are shared ways of practicing religion. The study highlights some of the elements of therapeutic religion, but also notes the tensions. Specifically, the study underscores how communities that permit and encourage self-expressions and experimentations may contribute to an appearance of "messiness," contradictions, chaos, and an appearance of excessive freedom at times.

That is to say, while therapeutic societies strive to equip individuals with "psychological capital," by giving people the license to both self-express and self-affirm, the culture of some of these emerging societies inadvertently may lead to certain excesses. Notably, this case study finds that the therapeutic ethic that characterizes one congregation has enabled some freedoms that are otherwise disallowed in traditional congregations. The visibility and regularity of certain behaviors, along with the permissive—indeed, sometimes graphic—sermon language, call attention to some of these excesses.

But this is not to say that this congregation disregards conventional norms altogether, or that therapy is used simply as an excuse for behavioral excesses. Rather, this study suggests that, in spite of the occasional "messiness" that may arise, therapeutic societies that serve marginalized and traumatized populations necessarily need to expand their functions. For religious organizations, this requires that the congregation integrate diverse functions (i.e., the therapeutic functions) into its religious repertoire. This is particularly the case if the immediate goal of the congregation is to eliminate human suffering, in which case a distinctly therapeutic and highly experimental form of religion may be pivotal in helping to reintegrate the wounded back into the community folds.

THE THERAPEUTIC ETHIC: A LITERATURE REVIEW

There are two traditions of individualism in the American context. The first is couched in terms of economic and material success, particularly when it results from ascetic behaviors. The second tradition of individualism refers to an inward feeling of freedom, comfort, and a self-perceived "authenticity that grounds our self-approval."[41] This latter tradition, termed expressive individualism or the "therapeutic ethic," emphasizes self-expression, uniqueness, autonomy, self-fulfillment, personal growth, and the search for an "authentic" self.[42, 43]

Scholars tend to view the therapeutic ethic critically, or at least ambivalently. Because the therapeutic ethic emphasizes dialogue and introspection, and its language and focus tend to center on "what feels good to me" or "what I can get,"[44] this ethic has been described as self-centered, narcissistic, selfish, and anti-community by scholars such as Robert Putnam,[45] Robert Bellah and the team from *Habits of the Heart*,[46] historian Christopher Lasch,[47] sociologist and cultural critic Philip Rieff,[48] among others. These critics believed (and feared) the therapeutic ethic would undermine collective sentiments and collective goals, eroding people's sense of duty to each other, and to the community at large. They predicted that as the therapeutic advanced, the focus on the private (the self) would replace a person's sense of public responsibility.

Rieff even went as far as to suggest that the therapeutic ethic would lead to the demise of western culture. According to Rieff, modern "psychological man" uses his community to enhance, rather than enrich, himself. With the use of therapy specifically, such an individual comes to focus on the present, and he unlearns ascetic traditions;[49] the weight is placed on instant, rather than deferred, gratification, and on impulse and release rather than self-control.

More generally, the needs of modern psychological man are said to trump communal needs, as the therapeutic ethic relegates the community subordinate to the individual. Thus, rather than contributing to the "stock" of social capital through civic commitments, the therapeutic ethic disintegrates it, or at least greatly loosens it.[50] This loosening of the civic structure caused by the "triumph of the therapeutic," in turn, increases social distance, contributing to the "the disuniting of America"[51] and, according to Rieff, ultimately the demise of western culture.[52]

This conventional perspective paints the therapeutic ethic in very broad strokes, portraying it as both all-consuming and with irreversible effects once it encroaches upon modern society. Yet, the fear that the therapeutic ethic will weaken communitarianism is not entirely off-base. Indeed, this point of concern has received empirical support in Greer and Roof's[53] study, which found an inverse relationship between privatized religion[54] and institutional religious loyalty.

Nonetheless, critics of the therapeutic ethic, while certainly justified in some of their critiques, fail to consider the complexities involved in self-expression. Moreover, the critics assume that few positive outcomes result from self-expression or therapy. This current study, therefore, calls for a more comprehensive analysis of the role of the therapeutic ethic, particularly as it pertains to multiply marginalized worshippers.

The conventional perspective of the therapeutic ethic assumes a dichotomy between the self and the other. Specifically, it is believed that self-interest (or self-love) necessarily comes at the expense of the interest of others (love for one's neighbors) and vice versa.[55] The propensity to polarize individualistic and community interests, however, assumes that people choose simply between private interests and the interests of the broad public good.[56] If we assume that maximizing the greatest good for the largest number is the ideal outcome, we might be inclined to prioritize communal interests. But such a choice obscures the benefits of individualism, and assumes that individualism and communitarianism are mutually exclusive, when they need not be.

While I suggest that the conventional perspective of the therapeutic ethic may be too narrow, the point of this paper is not to build a strawman out of Rieff's and others' critiques of the therapeutic ethic. Rather, this project argues for a reconsideration of the therapeutic ethic, which carries important and often unacknowledged implications. At the same time, I also draw attention to some of the real concerns and limitations of therapeutic societies.

RESEARCH METHODOLOGY:
THE CASE STUDY OF UNITY FELLOWSHIP CHURCH

This is a case study of Unity Fellowship Church, a small congregation in Los Angeles, California, whose congregants are gay, lesbian, bisexual, and transgendered (GLBT) African Americans.[57] This study comprises of field work, interviews, and content analysis of sermons. I disclosed my research intention to congregation members early on in the study, necessitated largely because of my outsider status as a non-religious, heterosexual, Asian-American woman. Given my outsider status, I was unable to participate in many support groups—notably the men's support groups, some HIV-support groups, and 12-step groups. I therefore supplemented the data with in-depth, face-to-face interviews. I further transcribed and analyzed the content of the sermons from services I attended during my three-and-a-half years in the field.

This study received approval from the Institutional Review Board at the University of Southern California. I obtained both verbal and written permission from Archbishop Bean to study his church and to disclose both his church's identity and his own identity. As the founder of Unity Fellowship Church and the Minority AIDS Project, Archbishop Bean is a well-known public figure. It therefore would have been extremely difficult, if not impossible, to conceal his identify. Most of the respondents consented to using their real names. Although I felt there was little risk of harm to the respondents, I ultimately felt it was best to err on the side of caution. Thus, although I have disclosed Archbishop Bean's identity, and have revealed the names of his church and outreach organization, I have used pseudonyms throughout this book for the remaining respondents.

The field work spanned over three years, from January 2002 to mid 2005. During this timeframe, I attended Sunday worship services, informally interacted with church members, and participated in religious classes, several church support groups, and a homeless outreach ministry. I also visited two daughter churches, one in San Diego and a second in Washington, DC.[58] I jotted down field notes when I could, but usually waited until I exited the field before recording my observations and thoughts, as note-taking would would have been far too conspicuous and intrusive.

The thirty-five interview respondents comprised of: ten clergy; twenty-four lay church members; and a single interview with the executive director of the church's outreach organization, the Minority AIDS Project (MAP).[59] Of the respondents, seventeen were men, fifteen were women, and three were male-to-female transgender individuals. The respondents ranged in age between twenty-five and sixty-four, with an average age of 46.4 years.[60] The respondents overwhelmingly identified as gay, lesbian, bisexual, or transgender.[61] In terms of religious backgrounds, most of the respondents had a firm foundation in Christianity beginning early in life. Most of the respondents came from a Baptist church or another black Protestant denomination.

A content analysis of church sermons supplemented the ethnographic data and interview data. Because African-American religions stress oral traditions,[62] analyzing the content of sermons became necessary. An examination of the religious discourse provides insight into the role of religion in modern society and how religious leaders communicate with their congregants,[63] I therefore transcribed verbatim the audio recordings of worship services that I attended during my three-and-a-half years in the field. Recurring themes and patterns in the sermons were noted.[64]

I intentionally collected data using multiple sources and multiple methods, in order to minimize the contaminating effects associated with possible researcher biases and differing worldviews.[65] In addition to triangulating the data, I attempted to ensure the internal validity of the data through member checking. This typically involved taking reports or specific descriptions or themes back to participants or informants and inquiring about the accuracy of certain events and descriptions.[66]

In all, I transcribed, coded line by line, and analyzed data generated from my attendance of sixty-one worship services, seventeen religious classes, twenty-one street outreach outings, nineteen support groups, and thirteen miscellaneous meetings, communications, and events. I also transcribed, coded, and analyzed the full transcripts from the thirty-five interviews. I electronically coded the data obtained from transcribed field notes, interview transcripts, and sermons using Atlas.ti 5.0.[67] Each field note, sermon, and interview transcript was examined separately, and as a part of the entire data set. Data from the interview transcripts were utilized as confirmation of both the salience and accuracy of themes I observed as a participant observer (e.g., themes found in the field notes). I assessed emerging themes, patterns, categories, and atypical responses and findings, using a grounded-theory approach.[68, 69, 70]

OUTLINE AND ARGUMENT OF THE BOOK

Chapter 2 provides portraits of Unity Fellowship Church, its founder, the Archbishop Carl Bean, and the congregation members. This chapter examines the history of the church and Archbishop Bean's influences. This chapter also examines the demographic characteristics and biographies of the church members, including their religious histories and how they found Unity Fellowship Church. Chapter 2 also highlights key rituals at Unity Fellowship Church. Important rituals for the Unity community include: testimonial service, affirmation, and, above all, the ritual of "hug and love." Therapeutic elements infuse the congregational practices. This is evident in both the embodied elements of some of the rituals, as well as in the therapeutic language that characterizes both the public and private messages (sermons and private talk).

Chapter 3 identifies some of the elements that have been missing in GLBT African-American worshippers' prior experiences in organized religion. The missing elements in their former congregations, as well as in their former understandings of religion, have shaped a more personalized, more therapeutic way of understanding religion.

Chapter 4 shifts from the organizational level to the micro level, and focuses on how congregation members adopt both the cultural (therapeutic) habits and styles of their church and combine it with their own lived experiences to make sense of religion, a personalized religion. This new religious form blends therapeutic language and new strategies of action that enable congregation members to integrate their religious and sexual identities. Exploring the dynamics by which theology and identities are entangled, and the processes congregation members use to disentangle conflicts between the two, this chapter examines specific strategies in which members of Unity Fellowship Church rely on as they construct new patterns of thinking and feeling in their attempts to reconcile the seemingly dissonance between religion and same-sex sexual orientation. Personalized religion, at least in the context of Unity Fellowship Church, is characterized by three distinct traits. First, the role, meaning, and meaningfulness of religion are open to interpretation. Second, religious identities are shaped by life experiences. Third, personalized religion, although individualized, is also a shared way of approaching religion.

Chapter 5 focuses on some of the freedoms and excesses that might arise with therapeutic religion. With respect to the congregation as the focus of this book, the excesses include overtly sexual behaviors, including cruising activities during worship services, provocative attire, and the occasional graphic sermon. A discussion of some of the unintended consequences of therapeutic religion is presented here. Cultural contributors of the excesses include: an individualized understanding of liberation theology; a therapeutic understanding of God; framing sin and sinning as suprapersonal; regarding the church as a hospital and medicalizing congregation members' behaviors; and an absence of a proscriptive language.

Chapter 6 highlights the ambivalence toward therapeutic religious forms, as represented through Wanda, a male-to-female transgender congregation member. On the one hand, Wanda very much needs many of the flexible rules and interpretations found at Unity. On the other hand, she is critical of those same flexible rules and interpretations. Wanda represents a congregation member who is still very much entrenched in traditional religion. She has not yet been able to extract herself from traditional forms of religion, including the more rigid rules and interpretations that characterize evangelical and more theologically conservative congregations. As a result, she is still in a liminal state, caught between two polarized religious forms, and she has yet to reconcile the two.

Chapter 7 underscores how, in spite of the perceived excesses at Unity Fellowship Church, the church and its members nonetheless conform to many mainstream norms, and the church pastor has articulated limits and boundaries. Indeed, congregation members themselves desire limits and boundaries, suggesting that this seemingly radically individualistic/therapeutic community is not simply self-indulgent.

Chapter 8 discusses why Unity Fellowship Church and therapeutic religion matter. For the respondents in this study, Unity provided not simply spiritual enlightenment but also enabled self-discovery and self-transformation. A religion that uncovers dirty secrets and taboo subjects, and affirms people with non-normative statuses, provides the pathway toward the liberation and reintegration of the spirit, the mind, and the body.

Chapter 9 concludes by reiterating the need for therapeutic religion, particularly for those in pain and those with a traumatic past. Pain demands a response of compassion, necessitating a counter-language of therapy or, in this case of Unity Fellowship Church members, therapeutic religion. The chapter stresses that although therapeutic religion is not perfect, and indeed it may give rise to openly sexual and other unconventional expressions, behaviors, and practices, the appearance of a certain "messiness" matters far less than the need for a religion that blends both theology and therapy. For the wounded and suffering spirits at Unity, who often have checkered pasts, therapeutic religion aims to reintegrate them back into a society.

NOTES

1. United States Census Bureau, "State and County QuickFacts," 2014, accessed June 2, 2014, http://quickfacts.census.gov/qfd/states/00000.html.
2. In terms of mode of transmission, the primary mode of HIV transmission among African-American men is sexual contact with other men. In 2010, African-American men who had same-sex sexual contact represented approximately 72 percent of new infections among all African-American men, with heterosexual contact the second leading mode of HIV transmission. In contrast, the primary mode of HIV transmission among African-American women was heterosexual contact (see Centers for Disease Control and Prevention 2005, 2014a, 2014b).
3. Centers for Disease Control and Prevention, "HIV among African Americans," 2014a, retrieved June 3, 2014, http://www.cdc.gov/hiv/risk/racialethnic/aa/facts/index.html.
4. Ibid.
5. Centers for Disease Control and Prevention, "Health Disparities in HIV/AIDS, Viral Hepatitis, STDs,and TB: African Americans/Blacks," 2014b, retrieved June 3, 2014, http://www.cdc.gov/nchhstp/healthdisparities/AfricanAmericans.html.
6. Office of Minority Health, U.S. Department of Health and Human Services, "HIV/AIDS and African Americans," 2013, retrieved June 3, 2014 http://minorityhealth.hhs.gov/templates/content.aspx?ID=3019.
7. Here, the term "black church" is used to differentiate denominations that are primarily African-American/black from white religious denominations. By no means does this imply that black churches are monolithic entities or denominations. Indeed, African-American/black churches are quite heterogeneous.
8. Cathy J. Cohen, *Boundaries of Blackness: AIDS and the Breakdown of Black Politics* (Chicago: University of Chicago Press, 1992).
9. Ibid.
10. Reginald Glenn Blaxton, "'Jesus Wept': Reflects on HIV Dis-ease and the Churches of Black Folk," in *Dangerous Liaisons: Blacks, Gays, and the Struggle for Equality*, ed. Eric Brandt (New York: The New Press, 1999), 109.

11.   Ronald Jeffrey Weatherford and Carole Boston Weatherford, *Somebody's Knocking at Your Door: AIDS and the African-American Church* (Binghamton, NY: Haworth Press, Inc., 1998).

12.   Kelly Brown Douglas, *Sexuality and the Black Church: A Womanist Perspective* (Maryknoll, NY: Orbis Books, 1999).

13.   Blaxton, "'Jesus Wept,'" 116–17.

14.   Cited from Gerard J. Stine, *AIDS update 1999* (Upper Saddle River, NJ: Prentice Hall, 1999), 398.

15.   Cited from Mary Beth Krouse, "Feminist Discursive Pivoting: Charting the Politics of AIDS," *Humanity & Society* 23, no. 1 (1999): 41.

16.   Vicki S. Freimuth, Sandra Crouse Quinn, Stephen B. Thomas, Galen Cole, Eric Zook, and Ted Duncan, "African Americans' Views on Research and the Tuskegee Syphilis Study," *Social Science & Medicine* 52, no. 5 (2001): 797–808.

17.   Kenneth J. Doka, *AIDS, Fear, and Society: Challenging the Dreaded Disease* (Bristol, PA: Taylor & Francis, 1997).

18.   Evelynn M. Hammonds, "Seeing AIDS: Race, Gender, and Representation," in *The Gender Politics of HIV/AIDS in Women*, eds. Nancy Goldstein and Jennifer Manlowe (New York: New York University Press, 1997), 115.

19.   Stephen Ellingson, Nelson Tebbe, Martha van Haitsma, and Edward O. Laumann, "Religion and the Politics of Sexuality," *Journal of Contemporary Ethnography* 30, no. 1 (2001): 3–55.

20.   Hammonds, "Seeing AIDS," 115.

21.   Gunnar Myrdal, *An American Dilemma: The Negro Problem and Modern Democracy* (reprint, New Brunswick, NJ: Transaction Publishers, [1944] 1996).

22.   Benjamin Mays and Joseph Nicholson, *The Negro's Church* (reprint, New York: Russell and Russell, [1933] 1969).

23.   Aldon D. Morris, *The Origins of the Civil Rights Movement: Black Communities Organizing for Change* (New York: Free Press, 1984).

24.   C. Eric Lincoln and Lawrence H. Mamiya, *The Black Church in the African American Experience* (Durham, NC: Duke University Press, 1990).

25.   Wyatt Tee Walker, "The Contemporary Black Church," In *The Black Church: A Community Resource,* eds. Dionne J. Jones and William H. Matthews (reprint, Washington, D.C.: Institute for Urban Affairs and Research, Howard University, [1976] 1977), 36.

26.   Patricia Hill Collins, *Black Feminist Thought: Knowledge, Consciousness, and the Politics of Empowerment*, 2nd ed. (New York: Routledge, 2000), 111.

27.   Howard Thurman, "The Anatomy of Segregation and Ground of Hope," in *African American Religious History: A Documentary Witness*, 2nd ed., ed. Milton C. Sernett (reprint, Durham, NC: Duke University Press, [1965] 1999), 548–54.

28.   Walker, "Contemporary Black Church."

29.   Blaxton, "'Jesus Wept,'" 111.

30.   Nick Freudenberg, "Health Promotion in the City: A Review of Current Practice and Future Prospects in the United States," *Annual Review of Public Health* 21 (2000): 491.

31.   Ibid.

32.   Peter L. Berger, *The Sacred Canopy: Elements of a Sociological Theory of Religion* (New York: Anchor Books, 1969).

33.   Omar M. McRoberts, *Streets of Glory: Church and Community in a Black Urban Neighborhood* (Chicago: University of Chicago Press, 2003).

34.   Marla F. Frederick, *Between Sundays: Black Women and Everyday Struggles of Faith* (Berkeley, CA: University of California Press, 2003).

35.   Irene Taviss Thomson, "The Theory That Won't Die: From Mass Society to the Decline of Social Capital," *Sociological Forum* 20, no. 3 (2005): 421–48.

36.   Paul Lichterman, *The Search for Political Community: American Activists Reinventing Commitment* (New York: Cambridge University Press, 1996).

37.   Robert N. Bellah, Richard Madsen, William M. Sullivan, Ann Swidler, and Steven M. Tipton, *Habits of the Heart: Individualism and Commitment in American Life* (reprint, Berkeley: University of California Press, [1985] 1996).

38. Christopher Lasch, *The Culture of Narcissism: American Life in an Age of Diminishing Expectations* (New York: W.W. Norton & Company, 1979).

39. Philip Rieff, *The Triumph of the Therapeutic: Uses of Faith After Freud* (reprint, Chicago: University of Chicago Press, [1966] 1987).

40. Pamela Leong, "Religion, Flesh, and Blood: Re-creating Religious Culture in the Context of HIV/AIDS," *Sociology of Religion* 67, no. 3 (2006): 295–311.

41. Bellah et al., *Habits of the Heart*, 79.

42. Thomson, "The Theory That Won't Die," 439.

43. Lichterman, *Search for Political Community*, 5–6.

44. Nina Eliasoph and Paul Lichterman, "Culture in Interaction," *American Journal of Sociology* 108, no. 4 (2003): 742.

45. Robert D. Putnam, *Bowling Alone: The Collapse and Revival of American Community* (New York: Simon & Schuster, 2000).

46. Bellah et al., *Habits of the Heart*.

47. Lasch, *Culture of Narcissism*.

48. Rieff, *Triumph of the Therapeutic*.

49. Ibid., 53–54.

50. Thomson, "The Theory That Won't Die," 441–42.

51. Arthur M. Schlesinger, Jr., *The Disuniting of America* (New York: H. H. Norton, 1992).

52. Rieff, *Triumph of the Therapeutic*, xv.

53. Bruce A. Greer and Wade Clark Roof, "'Desperately Seeking Sheila': Locating Religious Privatism in American Society," *Journal for the Scientific Study of Religion* 31, no. 3 (1992): 346–52.

54. Greer and Roof define "privatized religion" as "highly subjective, deeply personal form of religion" (p. 347). Others might define privatized religion as highly individualized and self-defined religion, ala "Sheilaism" (see Bellah et al., *Habits of the Heart*).

55. Stephen Pope, "Expressive Individualism and True Self-Love: A Thomistic Perspective," *The Journal of Religion* 71, no. 3 (1991): 385–86.

56. Lichterman, *Search for Political Community*, 10–11.

57. Funding for this study came from the Pew Charitable Trusts Dissertation Grant for Research on Religion, obtained through the Center for Religion and Civic Culture at the University of Southern California. The Department of Sociology at USC provided additional seed money.

58. The "Unity Fellowship Church Movement" comprises a network of twelve churches across the United States at the time of the study. The Los Angeles church is the mother church. I visited daughter churches in San Diego and Washington, DC.

59. Most of the interviews were obtained through a combination of purposive and snowball sampling. Each respondent was paid $20 for the interview, regardless of interview length. The interviews ranged from 1.67 hours to 7.25 hours. The interviews contained clusters of questions that focused on the following broad areas: 1) member background and religious history; 2) the church history and church characteristics; 3) church leadership; 4) church assessment; and 5) religious beliefs and practices.

60. The majority of the respondents were over forty.

61. One clergy identified as heterosexual.

62. Douglas, *Sexuality and the Black Church*.

63. Kimon Howland Sargeant, *Seeker Churches: Promoting Traditional Religion in Nontraditional Ways* (New Brunswick, NJ: Rutgers University Press, 2000), 78.

64. Audio recordings of worship services were made available by the church for a small fee. I transcribed the recordings verbatim.

65. Robert M. Emerson, *Contemporary Field Research: Perspectives and Formulations*, 2nd ed. (Prospect Heights, IL: Waveland Press, Inc. 2001).

66. John W. Creswell, *Research Design: Qualitative, Quantitative, and Mixed Methods Approaches*, 2nd ed. (Thousand Oaks, CA: Sage Publications, 2003).

67. Thomas Muhr, *User's Manual for ATLAS.ti 5.0* (ATLAS.ti Scientific Software Development GmbH, Berlin, 2004).

68.   Barney G. Glaser and Anselm L. Strauss, *The Discovery of Grounded Theory: Strategies for Qualitative Research* (New York: Aldine de Gruyter, 1967).

69.   Anselm Strauss and Juliet Corbin, *Basics of Qualitative Research: Grounded Theory Procedures and Techniques* (Newbury Park, CA: Sage Publications, 1990).

70.   Although the data collection and analysis in this study conform to most of the strategies attributed to grounded theory, I did not adhere rigidly to the approach outlined by Glaser and Strauss (1967), Strauss and Corbin (1990), and Emerson (2001). Given the sheer length of the interviews and sermons, and the ensuring transcription time, the bulk of the analysis came after data collection, although analysis also occurred as I analyzed, memoed, and coded my field notes. The process was often cyclical, wherein I would review literatures, collect, code, and analyze the data, find emerging themes and relationships between them, revise the analysis, and return to the literature.

Chapter Two

A Portrait of Unity Fellowship Church

ARCHBISHOP BEAN AND THE FOUNDING OF THE CHURCH

Unity Fellowship Church[1] is a Christian, nondenominational congregation in South Los Angeles with a predominantly African-American base. The church was founded in 1982 by an openly gay pastor, Reverend Carl Bean (now Archbishop), for primarily openly gay and lesbian African Americans. The first meetings were "rap groups" held in the private residence of some of the members, including Reverend Bean himself. Thereafter, the group met in more public settings. The first public worship service was held at the Cockatoo Inn in Inglewood, California. The services then relocated to the Ebony Showcase Theater in Los Angeles, considered as one of the hearts of the black Southern California community. In 1988, the church moved to the current location on West Jefferson Boulevard in Los Angeles.

The church received its non-profit status in 1985. In 1990, the movement—the Unity Fellowship Church Movement—was registered as a nonpartisan, non-profit organization.[2] Presently, the Unity Fellowship Church Movement comprises a network of churches across the United States.[3]

In 1985, Reverend Bean founded the Minority AIDS Project (MAP), the church's first outreach. According to the church and MAP websites, as well as organizational literatures, MAP is the first community-based HIV/AIDS organization in the United States that was established and maintained by people of color. This grassroots organization provides a broad range of HIV-related services for both clients and community members.[4]

Reverend Bean's work with those afflicted with AIDS preceded the founding of both his church and MAP, and the services that MAP initially provided simply comprised of what Reverend Bean was already doing: visiting the ailing in hospitals. Frequently, social workers would contact Reverend Bean to alert him of another AIDS-stricken patient. Often, the patients were racial minorities. While visiting the ailing, Bean also communicated with the social workers, the doctors and other health care staff, and the families of the afflicted. He observed that during his visits, the collar somehow dampened the anger and fears. As Bean himself described it, the idea of the symbol of a clergyperson seemed to soften the blow, or "stopped the anger at the kid or the child of the parent. . . . It changed the dynamic of, maybe, blame or sin."[5]

As Unity and MAP evolved, so, too, did a more formal system of organization. Since Reverend Bean was interacting and providing spiritual and counseling services for a "group of faithful people with AIDS from every discipline within Christendom you can imagine," he knew that he and his staff would need to use religious language that was comfortable for all of them. That included religious titles. Although the black Protestant denominations technically lack an official archbishop, black Protestants, according to Archbishop Bean, use "other words" in place of "archbishop." This includes the title "presiding bishop" and "presiding prelate."

Archbishop Bean noted that whenever he found himself in an ecumenical setting, people would refer to him as "the founder of the Unity Fellowship Church Movement, the Archbishop, or the Presiding Bishop of the Unity Fellowship Church. . . . The language just kept coming at me." Because people kept asking for titles, Bean therefore felt that having official religious titles were necessary. He consulted his church board. The board members had all come from the Baptist tradition or from other black denominations, and were comfortable with using the language around bishops. Hence, the Unity Fellowship Church network now involves an organizational system that is mostly similar to the black Protestant traditions, with tweaks here and there.

Both Archbishop Bean and Reverend Linda, in separate interviews with them, mentioned that Bean needed to sidestep the usual ordination process in order to gain his religious credentials. According to GLBT.com, Archbishop Bean at one point was a member of the Metropolitan Community Church (MCC) soon after his arrival in California in the 1970s.[6] The website also noted that Bean was enrolled in the MCC's Samaritan College in 1978 and was ordained as a minister four years later.[7]

It is likely that Archbishop Bean was at least partly inspired by the leadership of Troy Perry and the Universal Fellowship of Metropolitan Community Churches.[8] Certainly, there are similarities between Unity Fellowship Church and the MCC churches. Both are gay-affirming, and at both congregations the theological image of God is a benevolent, loving God that affirms gay men and women.[9] However, the respondent interviews seem to suggest that Unity differs from MCC not only in terms of its racial and ethnic constituency (Unity's African-American constituency versus the predominantly white congregations of the MCC churches) but in its religious rituals (Unity's black religious traditions versus MCC's "more Catholic" or "more traditional" elements, according to one respondent) and in the level of reliance on therapy. Hence, we see that Archbishop Bean clearly has drawn from his own background, particularly in terms of incorporating the black religious tradition and infusing therapy into church rituals, but he, too, has borrowed from the MCC. This is especially notable in terms of the reliance on liberation theology to integrate GLBT people into the religious folds and, more broadly, MCC's integrationist goals.

But there are still other similarities, including the origins of both churches. Both churches started out as a small group, in the founder's residence. From there, membership expanded, and so did the church space. Both congregations (and movements) arose and evolved during auspicious periods: the MCC, in the late 1960s, at the height of the gay liberation movement; and Unity Fellowship Church, in the early 1980s, at the height of the AIDS epidemic. In 1970, Troy Perry, the founder of the MCC churches, fasted for ten days on the steps of the Los Angeles Federal Building in order to publicize the demand for legal rights for gay men and women.[10] In the 1980s, Archbishop Bean staged a fast to protest the unequal funding allotted to community-based AIDS organizations. Both leaders are very charismatic, with a large following.[11]

Surely, gay-affirming congregations share some common attributes—notably, a benevolent, loving God who loves gays just as He loves heterosexuals, as well as a more expansive and inclusive theology. But if Archbishop Bean were previously a member of an MCC, borrowing MCC elements is almost inevitable. It does appear that many MCC elements are present at Unity, but Unity Fellowship Church is not simply a copy of MCC but for a black constituency.

Melissa Wilcox, who studied the Metropolitan Community Churches, described the MCC as a hybrid organization in that it blends old American traditions with new ones. In particular, she notes that the MCC retains some of the more conservative elements of religion—notably, in its affirmation of charismatic gifts, certain theological elements, and its emphasis on evangelism and its Pentecostal roots[12] —while simultaneously incorporating "radical" elements that celebrate and affirm GLBT people. Unity Fellowship Church is a hybrid organization, too. It is hybrid not only in that it draws from both traditional and modern sources, but it also draws from both religious and secular (therapeutic) elements, and it does so in ways that arguably are far more radical than the MCC churches.

What distinguishes Unity Fellowship Church from the Metropolitan Community Churches is, first, the congregation's constituency (primarily African American versus primarily white) and, second, the reliance on therapy to address a population that is marginalized, wounded, and scarred. To achieve this, however, requires a benevolent God who loves unconditionally, regardless of the person's social statuses. A therapeutic reframing of God, then, requires a God that is perhaps much more expansive than James Cone's[13] God, and even more expansive than the Metropolitan Community Church's God. The God at Unity necessarily must love even the most transgressive person.

Similarly, the theology at Unity—liberation theology—is therapeutically oriented. This is in spite of the fact that Archbishop Bean interprets liberation theology in collectivist terms, emphasizing class and race consciousness, social organization, and social change—consistent with liberation theology's original meaning. However, because of the heavy infusion of the therapeutic ethic at Unity, congregation members at Unity have interpreted liberation theology a bit differently than what was intended for either Latin-American, Roman-Catholic liberation theology[14] or James Cone's[15] black liberation theology.

Specifically, while Archbishop Bean couches liberation theology broadly as "freedom from oppression," and he relies mostly on a rights-and-social-justice language, at the same time his emphasis on liberating the GLBT population from shame, guilt, and other forms of internal distress enables his congregants to interpret "liberation theology" in more individualistic, therapeutic terms. Commonly, congregation members at Unity viewed liberation theology as the ability to interpret scripture as one sees fit, without having other people's demands and expectations imposed upon them. Other congregation members felt liberation theology simply meant a more inclusive and more expansive way of thinking. Still, other congregation members felt that liberation theology meant interpreting the Bible in non-oppressive ways, or at least understanding the context of when the Bible was written, in order to understand that meanings have changed over time. Others felt that liberation theology simply implied a God that "loves me just the way I am."

Although there are more expansive ways to interpret religion at Unity Fellowship Church, Archbishop Bean nonetheless has retained traditions that are important to his congregants, many of whom have deep religious roots. Specifically, black religious elements—and Baptist elements in particular—are conspicuous. Worship services at Unity Fellowship Church weave Baptist elements (for instance, the call-and-response style of preaching, singing, dancing, and other embodied rituals), social justice teachings, and therapy—three fundamental elements of the black Christian tradition. The sermons also are consistent with traditional religious teachings, as they stress God's benevolence and unconditional love, Jesus' identification with the least of them, and various social justice issues. In this respect, Unity Fellowship Church is very much in line with traditional black religions, in spite of housing members with vastly different demographic characteristics than those at mainline black congregations.

Overall, the therapeutic elements at Unity appear consistent with black religion. The difference, however, is the degree to which therapy is prioritized at Unity. Given their wounded states, congregation members at Unity yearn for, and expect, therapy. Archbishop Bean has answered accordingly, and he has infused therapy throughout religious services and congregational life. In worship services, there is an emphasis on emotional healing and the psychological well-being of individuals. The message that encourages that congregants "love themselves" is reiterated with great frequency.

THE CHURCH MEMBERS

Archbishop Bean remains in command of the mother church in Los Angeles, and of the Unity Fellowship Church movement. During the period in which I engaged in field work and interviews, there were four reverends, at least five ministers, and a handful of deacons at the mother church.[16] At the time of my data collection, one clergy estimated that there were approximately 150 to 200 active church members in the mother church alone.

In terms of the demographic characteristics of the congregation members, congregation members are primarily gay, lesbian, bisexual, and transgendered African Americans. Many of the church members are economically at the margins, with many unemployed or underemployed and/or on disability. The education level of members varies across the spectrum, from illiterate to limited education to some college-level work to post-graduate work, but most church members have at least a high school degree.

Many congregation members are in recovery, recovering from alcohol, drug, and/or sex addiction. Some have participated in survival sex at some point in their lives, mostly to finance a costly drug habit, while others are survivors of sexual violence and abuse. Violence, incarceration, and homelessness are not uncommon histories. Some of the members even continue to move in and out of the prison system. In addition, a considerable number of congregation members have mental illnesses and are on some sort of psychotropic medication, and one clergy estimates that between 20–50 percent of the congregation is HIV-positive.

The most typical biography of a congregant at Unity Fellowship Church, however, includes the experience with the stigma associated with being both black and gay and/or HIV-positive. Some of the interview respondents detailed histories of ostracism from family, although others also described very supportive and loving families.

Many respondents also described encountering homophobic and fear-mongering churches at least at one point in their lives. As Kambo described it:

[T]here's a lot of people out there that are hurting from the messages that they got in traditional churches. I mean it causes deep wounds. It really causes a lot of pain to think that God doesn't love you or that you're going to hell or that you're an abomination. . . .

Candy concurred, adding:

[A]s soon as they [the black churches] think you're . . . gay, they really ostracize you. They kinda make you feel like you're the scum of the earth. And they kinda point you out. . . . It's okay if you're gay and directing the choir, [b]ut as long as it's not talked about and not [in the] open . . .

Again and again, the interview respondents underscored the role of religious denouncements on the self-esteem of congregation members. A few respondents even made it a special point to highlight the behavioral effects of religious condemnation. Jones, for instance, articulated how the religious alienation experienced by men who have sex with other men was forcing them to "go on the down low,"[17] thereby contributing to the spread of HIV/AIDS. Samuel similarly subscribed to the notion that low self-worth leads to self-hate, in turn leading toward a path of self-destruction in which the person invariably causes harm to others. As Samuel summarized, "See, if you believe that the God you serve doesn't like you . . . the real message . . . that you're receiving [is] that [you're] not worth anything." In general, the general sentiment among the respondents was that there was a paradox inherent in the messages disseminated from the pulpit of most congregations. This was summed up by Jackie, who described the churches as preaching and teaching love, but "they demonstrate something else."

Some of the respondents in this study suggested that the religious leaders and the culture of organized religion tend to attribute defects, deficiencies, and deviance to the individual themselves, while failing to acknowledge institutional contributors to people's non-normative lives. The institutionalized expressions of homophobia and other forms of hate, however, have forced many of the people at Unity Fellowship Church to withdraw from their previous congregations, and to seek out congregations that will affirm them for who they are: gay and lesbian, African-American Christians.

Most of the congregation members at Unity had a firm foundation in Christianity beginning early in life. Most of the congregation members came from a Baptist church or another black Protestant denomination. In terms of the church members I interviewed,[18] nineteen respondents indicated a Baptist upbringing. Three respondents noted a Catholic upbringing, and three indicated an affiliation with a Church of God in Christ (COGIC).[19] Two respondents came from a Methodist background. Two respondents indicated simply a generic "Christian" upbringing, either non-denominational or the denomination was not indicated. Two respondents were raised in a Holiness church.

At least four respondents indicated being exposed to two or more religious traditions simultaneously.[20] A single respondent each indicated an affiliation with the following denominations: Apostolic, Christian Science, and Episcopalian. One respondent indicated no religious affiliation whatsoever in his early childhood years.

Based on the respondent descriptions of alienating, if not hateful, religious messages, it should not be surprising that a number of the respondents departed their childhood congregations and shopped around for a new place to worship. However, for some of the respondents, their religious foundation was deeply rooted in them; it was not something they could discard easily. Many of the respondents expressed disenchantment with the religious organization to which they were members during their upbringing. Many of these respondents exited the religious organization altogether, even if only temporarily. Countervailing tendencies seemed to pull them back from isolation, however, thrusting them back into a religious society.

For congregation members at Unity Fellowship Church, religion is very much a part of their life. Indeed, some of the respondents expressed a longing for the spiritual experience that was long a part of their culture and long a part of their life, but they wanted something more: They wanted and needed a spiritual life that affirmed them in totality. Kambo, for one, joined Unity Fellowship Church because he was looking for a new way of understanding God. "That was my most basic thing," he stated, but then added, "I definitely wanted to be affirmed. I didn't want to be a hypocrite anymore [and be in the closet]." An authentic religion and authentic church for Kambo meant that he could be openly homosexual. It meant that he did not have to check his homosexuality at the church doors, nor did he have to be a "hypocrite" and preach against homosexuality while secretly engaging in homosexual acts behind closed doors.

Pushed out of their churches, congregation members at Unity described a period of church hopping and church shopping as they struggled to harmonize their sexual identity with their religious identity. Separated from their previous religious anchor, they also were not linked to new ones. Thus, many congregation members at Unity Fellowship Church, between the period they attended their family church and Unity, experienced a period of liminalness in which they were neither here nor there. In this period, they church hopped and church shopped.

Fourteen respondents in this study flirted with other denominations, church-hopping, and visiting multiple churches. Among these churches included African Methodist Episcopalian, Apostolic, Church of God and Christ, and non-denominational Christian congregations. One respondent attended a Unitarian congregation that he described as new-agey, and that focused more on nature and the earth than on religion. Another respondent attended both Unity Fellowship Church and a synagogue concurrently. Two other respondents simply indicated they attended "spiritual" churches during their church-seeking period.

At least ten respondents visited gay-affirming churches, with the Metropolitan Community Churches (MCC) most cited by the respondents. The MCC is an international denomination that fosters the beliefs that homosexuality is a gift from God and that God makes people diverse to fulfill divine purposes. MCC's theology posits that Christians should equally value all genders, sexual orientations, races, and ethnicities. [21]

In many ways, the beliefs of the Metropolitan Community Churches are in line with those of Unity Fellowship Church. The differences between the two churches, however, are not small. Foremost, congregation members at Unity Fellowship Church who have attended an MCC church consistently cited the racial and ethnic homogeneity of the MCC churches: They are overwhelmingly white. This point is confirmed by Rodriguez and Ouellette, [22] who maintain that while the churches in the MCC network are considered ethnically diverse, it is still majority white.

Ramona, who describes herself as "always been Baptist," chronicled her religious trajectory. She grew up in her mother's Pentecostal church, but "became my own" when she was older. She stated that she had to exit her church because "they condemned me [as a homosexual] in the church . . . [and] at that time, I think that AIDS had just come out and it really tainted my views on religion." But even after dissociating herself from her church, and coming out, she held steadfast to her God. She explained, "I always had God in my heart and I never really sat down and decided on organized religion." She visited a Metropolitan Community Church, a non-denominational, gay-affirming congregation, but did not identify with what she felt were "Catholic elements" at this particular church. She explained, "I know me and what I'm comfortable with." Going to another Baptist church or even a non-Baptist church that was gay-affirming but that had culturally discordant elements, however, was "not me. I don't force it. . . . I'm not into that. It just wasn't me." Thus, for Ramona, being a part of a gay-affirming church was important, but that was not enough. She needed to return to her African-American religious roots.

Kambo, too, spoke of the need to return to black religion after experimenting with other religious forms. He dabbled in assorted religions, beginning with Eastern religion "'cause I was feeling a whole thing about mysticism and stuff like that." He then "started seeing things" in sophism, Islam, Buddhism, and Taoism. He explained that he felt like he needed to create his own religion, because the religion in which he was raised was simply "not working," but he did not have any guidance or direction with respect to which religion to turn. He turned to popular culture at one point, although not intentionally doing so. He confessed that a book about the Broadway play *A Chorus Line*, in which a couple characters who were gay and became Buddhists, convinced him at least to explore Buddhism. Yet, throughout this period of religious experimentation, Kambo just "couldn't get away from the tradition of being in church . . . in the traditional black church," because this was what he grew up with, and traditional black religion was something he did not want to lose or give up, as it was a part of his identity. He found what he wanted and needed at Unity Fellowship Church from the outset.

Jarvis pointed out the acute divisions between the predominantly white congregations and the predominantly black congregations, and noted how this division was apparent even among the gay-affirming congregations. He described the cultural differences that, on the one hand, require separate congregations that culturally affirm the population that make up the congregation. He explained, for instance, that black congregations have "a different style of [religious] teaching," and described people of color as "much louder" and "their services are much longer." These are some of the elements of traditional black religion, elements unfamiliar to many non-black worshippers and elements that are absent at primarily gay-affirming white congregations, including the MCC churches.

But there were other differences between the gay-affirming congregations beyond differences in racial constituencies. Minister Pepper highlighted the differences in the sermon content, noting that even at a gay-affirming congregation such as the MCC, she never heard messages that explicitly articulated that it was "okay" to be gay, bisexual, transgender, and so forth. She described the MCC worship services as "more of a regular service," in that it lacked any messages about homosexuality—at least not at the services she attended. The MCC services she attended simply focused on the Bible, and "sang the same [religious] songs." Candy concurred with this assessment, noting that even the times when she visited some of the MCC churches, she never heard messages that proclaimed that "God made you just the way you are," and that it's okay to be "gay or lesbian or bi or trans or this or that . . . or the other." This suggests that for black GLBT worshippers, there is a need to explicitly affirm their GLBT status.

There were other cultural differences noted. Safiyah went as far as to describe MCC as "conservative" and "staid," noting that men in drag were never found at the MCC churches. In other words, it appears that the MCC worship services conform to what one would expect of a worship service, despite the fact that gay men and women comprise the congregation. Absent, however, are the flamboyant elements stereotypically associated with the gay lifestyle: the over-the-top attire, the cross-gendered behaviors, and so forth. In other words, Safiyah was alluding to gay men and women's need to be openly self-expressive, including in their attire and styles, rather than conform to conservative norms.

In general, the interview data revealed that having a gay-affirming congregation is important, but this element alone was not enough to permanently draw members into the church. Also needed was an explicit discussion of GLBT issues from the pulpit, as well as explicit affirmations of church members' GLBT status. Finally, for people with deep religious roots in the black religious tradition, the congregation has to be rooted in African-American religious traditions. That is, an "authentic" church for GBLT African Americans is not only gay-affirming but Afrocentric; it must affirm the person wholly, and in no uncertain terms.

CHURCH RITUALS

Worship services at Unity Fellowship Church partly reflect Archbishop Bean's religious influences: There are elements from the southern civil rights movements (anti-institutionalism, social-justice rhetoric, etc.) and elements from the black Baptist tradition, both reflecting his childhood socialization influences. What is distinct about Unity Fellowship Church's culture, however, is that Archbishop Bean has pieced together different elements to form a distinct religious style and culture that maintains some of the traditional black religious elements, but with a twist: It is more personalized and more flexible, and there is a higher level of emotional involvement in worship service and church life.

Samuel described the "freedom of spirit" he observed at Unity as "totally different than some other churches." This "freedom of spirit" is particularly evident in the embodied aspects of worship services. While the Baptist influences in the worship rituals are present, Unity is unlike the church in Baltimore in which a young Carl Bean was raised. Archbishop Bean's childhood church was upwardly mobile and sophisticated, and there was an absence of embodied rituals. As Archbishop Bean described it, there was "no hand-clapping, no hollering out. . . . We sang anthems, we had a pipe organ, we held sheet music and sang by note. It was . . . I came from something very different from what I see [at Unity]."

Archbishop Bean acknowledged that it would not have worked had he run Unity Fellowship Church in the style of the traditional black churches. Having been raised in a traditional religious structure, which he characterized as structured, methodical, and rigid, Bean admitted that he himself would have been comfortable in such an environment, but knew that style would not work for his congregants. Services at traditional black churches were held at eleven a.m. on the dot every Sunday. There were far too many rules, and it was too structured. It was also too stern. Affective displays were disallowed, as was "shouting back" to the preacher. Such styles and rituals likely would not resonate with the congregants at Unity Fellowship Church, however, because they would have required that congregants suppress their lived experiences, including their most painful experiences, and what they were experiencing and feeling at that moment.

Archbishop Bean explained that much of the theology he learned was taught through people's personal experiences, and he believes that one must incorporate personal experiences into one's religion or spirituality. In fact, he indicates that he tells congregation members, "Your experiential walk is the key to your spirituality. . . . Whatever your experience has been, your experiential walk is what will give you assurance around the presence around an almighty father or mother."

Integrating the experiences of Unity Fellowship Church members, however, requires flexibility and creativity. Indeed, from the church's infancy, when it was simply an informal study group, Bean allowed the group to develop in accordance to the needs of the people, rather than try to prescribe it with his own religious views, experiences, and demands. Similarly, worship services and other church activities also flow around congregation members' needs. On occasions, for instance, Archbishop Bean may deviate from worship routines because he senses certain congregation members suffering and in despair. On those occasions, instead of preaching in a lecture style, Archbishop Bean may, instead, preach using song. On other occasions, he may instruct the congregants to interact with one another, usually through verbal affirmations or embraces. The choice of musical selection also may change at the spur of the moment, depending on the congregants' moods and affective states, something to which Archbishop Bean seems to be very attune. On occasions, the music is quick-paced and upbeat, reflecting the joys and energy of the congregation; on other occasions, the tempo of the song is slow and melodic, reflecting their pain.

Given the backgrounds of Unity Fellowship Church members, it is not surprising that this congregation's form of religion is characterized by a therapeutic ethic that encourages the expression of the authentic, expressive self, and that demarcates the self as the center of authentic feelings and needs that must be uncovered, explored, and expressed.[23] For traumatized people, the need to express the self is particularly crucial. Archbishop Bean recognizes this point and has institutionalized various therapeutic practices in worship services and in church support groups. These practices include affective and embodied rituals that stress the affirmation of the whole person, that embolden participants to publicly disclose secrets, and that encourage members to unleash their emotions. Key rituals include: testimonials, affirmation; hug and love; and the embodied elements of worship services—the crying, shouting, and dancing—as well as the visual and verbal displays of "love."

Unity Fellowship Church's liberation theology primarily is inward-oriented, as its theology focuses more on the liberation of individuals from guilt and other distressful emotions. Archbishop Bean believes that liberation from guilt and shame necessarily involves the freedom to disclose secrets and the freedom to be honest. Indeed, it is Archbishop Bean's belief that concealing a part of oneself—particularly if it is a major status that shapes one's identity (e.g., sexual orientation)—creates significant internal turmoil. This, in turn, may give rise to the fear of others, self-hatred, and the hatred of others. Representing a safe place of healing, Unity gives its members "permission to be honest"[24] and allows its members to share secrets.

The testimonial service that precedes each worship service is one forum for the disclosures of secrets. In this portion of the service, congregation members openly disclose: their physical and emotional health statuses (including HIV status); problems with addictions; feelings of ambivalence about sexuality and HIV status; rejection and ostracism by family, friends, and employers; relationship difficulties; unemployment; financial insolvency; suicidal ideations; near-death experiences; and still other personal challenges.

Because a significant proportion of Unity's members are affected by HIV/AIDS, AIDS-related dialogue is common. During testimonial services, parishioners publicly proclaim their HIV status and detail their health care regimens. Conversations about T-cell count, dietary restrictions, weight loss, difficulty in mobility and difficulty in performing instrumental tasks of daily living, loss of bodily control and function, and physical pain are common. There are also personal testimonies about: feelings of ambivalence about sexuality and HIV status; rejection and ostracism by family, friends, and employers; relationship difficulties; substance abuse addiction; unemployment; financial insolvency; suicidal ideations; and near-death experiences.

Religious leaders themselves acknowledge their own HIV-positive status and, in doing so, normalize HIV/AIDS. They also openly discuss matters involving non-hetero sexualities. This is in stark contrast to the more mainstream faith communities, which, according to the respondents, tend to avoid matters involving sexuality altogether and which tend not to contest homophobia. In all, at Unity Fellowship Church, congregation members are not afraid to disclose personal secrets; indeed, they willingly address issues that other religious institutions avoid altogether.

Disclosing secrets is part of the healing process. Much like a twelve-step program, admitting that a problem exists is a necessary first step toward recovery. Being aware of the problem then enables a congregation member to better confront the problem. The awareness also allows the congregation members to examine him or herself in a more forthright manner, and to confront the problem realistically and honestly. Honesty means acceptance and admission of one's addictions and unhealthy behaviors.[25] For recovery groups, acknowledging that a problem exists is a first step—and a crucial step—to recovery and healing. Archbishop Bean and the clergy at Unity Fellowship Church acknowledge this pivotal step and, accordingly, attempt to facilitate the recovery process through testimonial services and various support groups.

But even the process of admission is not a quick or linear one. Shelly, for one, mustered the courage to openly disclose her positive-HIV status, although it required an eight-year "healing process" and the need to first "grow through a lot of stuff" before she was able to do so. She explained how challenging her HIV disclosure was for her:

> [I]n my world, there's not that many women . . . especially so-called studs [butch lesbians] . . . that would even admit to sleeping with men. . . . And having a brother that passed away from [AIDS] and understanding the way society looks upon this disease as a modern-date leprosy and a punishment from God . . . [E]ven though I was welcome and open and feel comfortable [at Unity], I couldn't say the words. I couldn't say the words. It was just a process. I was openly a drug addict . . . a recovering drug addict. Openly a prostitute. You know, I was so many things in my life and in my story that I told publicly at the podium, all over this land. But I couldn't say that . . . words. I just couldn't feel ostracized anymore . . . for being black, for being female, for being gay. [AIDS] was just one more burden that I just didn't . . . couldn't say. And once I said it, it was the most liberating thing that ever happened. See, that's why I said the church, in so many avenues, [has] been my friend. Yeah, has been my freedom.

Shelly's underscoring of "my freedom" is a nod to both Unity Fellowship Church's therapeutic ethic and its liberation ethic, which, in many ways, are really one and the same. Although it took her close to a decade, it was only through the support of a non-judgmental community was she able to unpack a secret that had burdened her for so long. Such a disclosure has set her free at last from shame, guilt, and fear, marking her first step to healing as an HIV-positive lesbian.

The purpose of therapy is emancipation. Therapy provides to the patient "unique freedoms" and access to "a final figure of authority."[26] Archbishop Bean represents this authority figure; he is Freud's therapist to the congregant-patient. Archbishop Bean listens, comprehends, and does not condemn. In return, his congregants tell all. Their obligation in the therapeutic relationship is to talk. And it is hard work, in part because the patients fear losing control.[27] And as many of the respondents have indicated to me, they also fear what others—what larger society—might think of them, and they frequently anticipated inhospitable treatment with the disclosure of certain secrets. Unity Fellowship Church, however, mitigates some of these fears, by first providing a safe and supportive space to disclose secrets, before congregants embark into the larger social world.

Affirmation is part of the healing process. Affirmation, in fact, is one of the most defining rituals at Unity Fellowship Church, according to the interview respondents. This ritual underscores the need to free oneself from guilt associated with having a non-hetero sexual orientation. Because the over-whelming majority of the congregation is GLBT, the clergy make it a special point to explicitly articulate the words "gay," "lesbian," "bisexual," and "transgender" at each Sunday worship service, and this is immediately fol-lowed by verbal proclamations that, regardless of one's sexual orientation, everyone is special and loved. Sexuality at Unity, thus, is normalized rather than problematized. Regardless of one's sexual orientation, sexuality is cele-brated and framed in the context of tolerance, self-acceptance, God, and love, rather than in moral or pathological terms. The following is a typical affirma-tion message.

> Whether you're hetero, whether you're asexual, it doesn't matter to Love. Just stand and be that which you are: God's perfect children. For you were created in perfection. Know that you were not an afterthought. Know that you were not an oops baby. Know that God never went back and recreated anything that God created. You are created the way you were supposed to be: in perfection, in the light of Love.

The clergy themselves frequently cite their own sexual orientations, and they stress that all sexual orientations are healthy, positive, and natural. This process of affirmation is a central ritual at Unity, and it provides an example of a ritual and tradition that underscores the uncompromising acceptance of differences.[28] It is Archbishop Bean's hope that through the repetition of affirmations, congregation members will then internalize the messages that their sexual orientations and other social statuses are normal and God-given, and that they are people who are worthy of God's support and love, and worthy of abundant life.

The ritual of affirmation is considered one of the most memorable and powerful rituals experienced by visitors, particularly first-time visitors. Wil-ma and Joy described their experiences. Wilma recalled, "I think when I heard, 'It's okay to be gay, transgender . . . ,' to just hear that. [And to hear], 'And God loves you,' those words right there . . . inspired me and just really hit me internally." Wilma's partner, Joy, indicated that she was so moved by the affirming messages that she became overcome with emotions. She stated, "I cried probably from the beginning until the end of service." Even Wanda, an outspoken critic of Unity, underscored the importance of Unity's affirma-tion. She stated, "[Affirmations] kind of confirmed you are who you are and in your wholeness and that you are okay who you are. And that really is a drawing point for me. That's what really drew me in."

Minister Macon explained how affirmation was an integral part of the church life, and that the repetition that "God loves you just the way you are" was especially crucial:

It's the same message. It's the same message because some people have been here five, six years and still don't get it. Some people. . . . It's mostly said for the newcomer, but it's like. . . . Well, when we talk, the message of hate has been said all your life, so when someone starts telling you that God loves you just the way you are one or two times, but you've heard 13, 14, 15, 20, 25 years of hate messages, just hearing that one or two times is not going to make a difference, but that's why the affirmation is included every Sunday.

The affirmations also resonate for Candy, who, I observed, still needed reminders that she is a person worthy of God's love and worthy of abundant living. When I interviewed Candy at her home, I noted all the post-it notes with affirmation messages taped on the walls of her dressing area. The presence of these affirmation notes suggested to me that, in spite of the frequent repetitions of affirmation at Unity, congregation members still needed reminders that they were worthy. The affirmations, in other words, could not—and should not—stop at the church doors.

Affirmation is followed immediately by "hug and love," a ritual in which congregants maneuver around the sanctuary and greet one other, regardless of degree of acquaintance, and verbalize to one another that "you are very special." But there is more to healing than simply verbal affirmations. There also is the healing power of touch. Indeed, sometimes all one needs is the healing touch—specifically, a simple but sincere hug. The hug-and-love ritual, thus, provides this healing element, as congregants both verbally affirm each other's specialness, and energy, life, and love flow from one person to another through the hug.

When I described to church outsiders this "hug-and-love" ritual, invariably I would hear snickers. To church outsiders, the ritual sounds corny and unserious, with little chance for success. But the interview respondents again and again noted to me how significant this ritual was; indeed, they described hug-and-love as one of the most powerful congregational rituals. This is true even among the long-time members, who may not "need" the hugs and may even prefer not to be hugged. For other members and for newcomers, however, the hug is crucial. As Raymond pointed out, "[Y]ou don't know what you may be going through or what somebody else might be going through. Just that hug . . . could make their day . . . for that moment right then and there. That's what they needed. They needed somebody to hug them." For marginalized populations such as those at Unity Fellowship Church, the ritual performativity of embraces and verbal affirmations may have profound psychological effects for "people who have not been touched all week, all month, or maybe all year." In fact, some of the worshippers at Unity go as far as to say, "That's the only time that I've ever gotten touched."

Hugging has become a pivotal part of Unity Fellowship Church, and hugging is another ritual that distinguishes Unity Fellowship Church from other congregations, where church members and church pastors tend not to hug. In fact, when I mentioned to Archbishop Bean that I just assumed pastors greet and embrace congregants, he laughed out loud and roared, "No, no, no [laughter]! That is so far beneath their dignity, oh! For a pastor to hug you? That's like pulling a gun on him. No. No, no, no." However, at his own church, Archbishop Bean felt hugging was crucial, particularly for those stricken with AIDS.

After observing firsthand how health care workers refused to come into contact with AIDS-stricken patients, Archbishop Bean knew it was necessary to help people become comfortable with those affected by AIDS, and to also let those stricken with AIDS know that they, too, were loved:

> I knew that in those days, people were very sick. You knew they had AIDS. . . . And they were, of course, coming to our church setting in droves. And I began to say, "How did you feel when you really wanted to know you were loved? Was it enough for someone to say it to you and you knew that the words just kind of didn't ring true? How did it feel when someone embraced you, like Grandma, when you knew it was love?" And they were scared. I said, now that's what we want to do [at Unity]. We don't care what happened all week, even this morning, but we want, here in this church, to say, "You are loved," and our words are going to be "You are very special." And when I finish this [the affirmation], I want you to get up and go around the room [and hug each other]. . . . I remember the first time—and I remember seeing what happened in that room as people said that to each other. And it became . . . I think one week I forgot it and they asked me, "Bishop, when we gonna do 'the special' [now referred to as affirmation and hug and love]?"

Early in the church's development, when worship services were confined to a small room at the building that now houses Minority AIDS Project, Archbishop Bean would hug parishioners as he came into the church in the precessional, and also when he exited the church in the recessional. Archbishop Bean would make it a special point to approach the person who "looked sickest" and would draw the individual into his arms. Thereafter, the junior clergy at Unity followed Archbishop Bean's example and also began to hug parishioners. Now, hugging is "a custom" at all of the Unity Fellowship Church congregations, and this ritual seems to have influenced other congregations as well.

But there was still a difference. I noted to Archbishop Bean that although "other churches" may hug, their hugs felt different, at least they did to me. But then, I was an outsider at pretty much all religious organizations, so the feeling of detachment might be expected. But even with my first visit at Unity Fellowship Church, the hugs felt real to me somehow; they were full-bodied hugs, with no hesitancy whatsoever in terms of touching a stranger. And direct eye contact was usually made. They felt genuine, rather than obligatory and forced. Archbishop Bean agreed with my assessment of the hugs I received at a mainline congregation that I visited. "It's not real embracing," he concurred, but then he tempered his evaluation by pointing out how the detached hugging is "very American!"

Archbishop Bean underscored how people need to be touched. He described how visitors to his church were initially afraid of hugging, because hugging seemed so foreign to them, as hugging was not a part of their lives. But then, these visitors, who would then become church members, would confess to him that once they felt the hugging at Unity, they "came looking for it," in spite of initially feeling hesitant.

Hugging, then, is therapeutic. This is because hugging and touching not only symbolize human connection, but it indicates acceptance. As Archbishop explained, "We want to know that we're welcome, and it's the most beautiful thing." He described how, as an entertainer, he would instruct audience members to approach the stage to shake his hands at the conclusion of a song. He recalled audience members literally running down the aisle to greet him. "They *run*," Archbishop Bean stated, explaining that this was because "people want a genuine touch and it means so much to them. So *much* to them!"

But the problem in American society is that physical contact between human beings may be misconstrued as sexual or inappropriate. As a result, people may be quite hesitant, even resistant, to hug. Archbishop Bean, however, acknowledges the need for humans to have genuine physical (non-sexual contact), and indicates that such contact "works." He declared, "It [hugging] works! And I don't know why we, as a species, are so afraid of what works. I don't know what that's about. We're so afraid of what we know works, you know? Across all lives, it works!"

At a religious class during Lent, one participant illustrated the cautious nature of Americans. Like many Americans, she, too, was wary of physical contact from strangers, as she expressed her discomfort with the hug-and-love ritual at Unity. She indicated that she was not used to people coming up to her—and complete strangers at that—and hugging her. But the participant then described how one woman came up to her and just gave her a "long, tight hug." The participant described feeling overwhelmed and emotional thereafter, as a result of a stranger reaching out to her and showing that she cared, and recognizing that the hugs from the congregants are not empty gestures but gestures of love.

Penny Edgell Becker[29] addressed a congregation's identity or culture ("who we are") in terms of "what we do" and "how we do things here." Unity Fellowship Church members represent a traumatized lot. It therefore makes much sense that the culture of Unity—that is, the "what we do" and "how we do things here"—are therapeutically oriented, with a focus on a "language of pain"[30] and the subsequent need for a language of therapy. Accordingly, at Unity Fellowship Church, therapy and religion are woven together. Indeed, the primacy of therapy is evident in not only the sermons, but also in the church rituals, worship music, and even activities and programs that are not exclusively religious. It is also evident in the way congregation members communicate to each other, both publicly and privately.

Therapeutic elements are prominent in the language of the church founder/pastor, clergy, and congregation members, not only in the public talk (the sermon), but in private talk, as well as in the course of the semi-structured, face-to-face interviews. In large part, these therapeutic-religious elements developed out of the unmistakable assumption that most congregation members have undergone some type of trauma. As a result, therapeutic language, ideas, and rituals are normative in this congregation.

This new-found religious freedom for self-expression, however, is not without its costs. A subsequent chapter focuses on some of the potential "excesses" of therapeutic religion, and their cultural contributors.

NOTES

1. Unity Fellowship Church is not a part of any national denomination or religious movement. It should therefore not be confused with the Unitarian Churches. Nor should it be confused with the Unity churches, the network of New Thought churches founded in the late 1800s by Charles and Myrtle Fillmore.

2. Unity Fellowship Church, "Unity Fellowship Church: History," Unity Fellowship Church of Christ Church, Inc., accessed January 31, 2007, http:// http://www.ufc-usa.org/history.htm.

3. According to the current website, the Unity Fellowship Church movement consists of fourteen daughter churches and the mother church (Unity Fellowship Church Los Angeles), for a current total of fifteen churches.

4. Because MAP spawned out of Unity, it is often difficult to disentangle the work of Unity and MAP. This task is made even more difficult because some of MAP's HIV programs are housed at Unity, and the programs are facilitated by MAP educators and consultants who are also church members and/or clergy.

5. But there was a more practical need for the visual (the collar). As Reverend Linda noted to me, in order for the public to take Unity Fellowship Church seriously as a legitimate religious organization, rather than a cult or a ritual, it was necessary that Carl Bean undergo an official ordination and wear the collar. The collar, she believed, served to remind the public that Bean is an authentic, respected religious leader.

6. This was a point of omission in my interview of both Archbishop Bean and Reverend Linda.

7. This was another point of omission in my interview with Archbishop Bean. There was also conflicting information with respect to where Archbishop Bean was ordained, and by whom.

8. Archbishop Bean actually noted briefly at one point in the interview that he was acquainted with Troy Perry. Another interview respondent acknowledged a relationship between Troy Perry and Archbishop Bean and mentioned that it was Perry himself who ordained Bean when Bean became archbishop of the Unity Fellowship Church movement in the late 1990s. The ordination took place in Washington, DC, and Archbishop Bean himself recalled that Perry *"might have"* given the sermon at his ordination.

9. Melissa M. Wilcox, "Of Markets and Missions: The Early History of the Universal Fellowship of Metropolitan Community Churches," *Religion and American Culture: A Journal of Interpretation* 11, no. 1 (2001): 83–108.

10. Ibid., 90.

11. There are other similarities between the two congregations and the leaders that I have not included here.

12. Melissa M. Wilcox, "Of Markets and Missions: The Early History of the Universal Fellowship of Metropolitan Community Churches," *Religion and American Culture: A Journal of Interpretation* 11, no. 1 (2001): 92.

13. James H. Cone, *A Black Theology of Liberation* (Maryknoll, NY: Orbis Books, 1990).

14. Christian Smith, *The Emergence of Liberation Theology: Radical Religion and Social Movement Theory* (Chicago: University of Chicago Press, 1990).

15. Cone, *A Black Theology of Liberation.*

16. Some of the clergy rose in rank during the timespan of this study. Ordination is in-house, usually occurring during the annual convocation in which members of the network of Unity Fellowship Churches meet.

17. "Down low" refers to a phenomenon in which men who do not identify as homosexual or bisexual engage in sex with other men, but otherwise lead a heterosexual-appearing life.

18. Here, I exclude the single interview of the executive director of the Minority AIDS Project.

19. Two of the respondents raised in the COGIC church were also Baptists simultaneously.

20. For example, Antoine indicated that he had a Catholic, Jehovah's Witness, and Southern Baptist upbringing, reflecting the religious affiliations of his grandfather, mother, and father, respectively.

21. Michelle Wolkomir, "Wrestling with the Angels of Meaning: The Revisionist Ideological Work of Gay and Ex-Gay Christian Men," *Symbolic Interaction* 24, no. 4 (2001): 409.

22. Eric M. Rodriguez and Suzanne C. Ouellette, "Gay and Lesbian Christians: Homosexual and Religious Identity Integration in the Members and Participants of a Gay-Positive Church," *Journal for the Scientific Study of Religion* 39, no. 3 (2000): 335.

23. Ann Swidler, *Talk of Love: How Culture Matters* (Chicago: University of Chicago Press, 2001), 146.

24. 3/10/04 Lent Service.

25. Gerald G. May, *Addiction and Grace* (New York: Harper & Row, 1988), 165.

26. Philip Rieff, *Freud: The Mind of the Moralist* (Garden City, NY: Anchor Books, 1961), 364.

27. Ibid.

28. While affirmation focuses on affirming GLBT status, GLBT affirmation is not the sole focus of the affirmation ritual. Indeed, the clergy also validate other identities (e.g., affirming one's identity as African American) in the affirmation message.

29. Penny Edgell Becker, *Congregations in Conflict: Cultural Models of Local Religious Life* (New York: Cambridge University Press, 1999).

30. Dawne Moon, *God, Sex, and Politics: Homosexuality and Everyday Theologies* (Chicago: University of Chicago Press, 2004).

Chapter Three

Wrestling with Religion and the Rise of Personalized Religion

The lives of congregation members at Unity Fellowship Church can be described, in many ways, as "unsettled." According to Ann Swidler,[1, 2] in such unsettled lives, people reorganize "strategies of action" or construct new ones, in order to adapt to the changes. Culture, in these cases, take a more explicit and more visible form, as the major life changes may require a reconsideration and transformation of culture, and new patterns of thinking and feeling come in contact and conflict with previous modes of action and experience.[3] During these unsettled cultural periods, people actively use culture to learn new ways of being. Some people construct new selves, while others establish families and other relationship forms.[4] Yet, in these unsettled periods, Swidler argued, people may still rely on their existing repertoire to organize action and make sense of the world around them.[5]

People who identify as gay, lesbian, bisexual, or transgender (GLBT) often are situated as social objects and placed in marginal or liminal states, with little sense of belonging in any community. GLBT worshippers are even further away from the mainstream, as they become uncemented from a firm religious foundation that became unfixed upon their GLBT identification. The sense of separation between one's identity and one's religious beliefs and teachings produces a sense of crisis, and disrupts the person's self-understanding of religion.

Rather than having a fixed religious identity (e.g., the religious affiliation of one's childhood religious upbringing), personalized forms of religion allow individuals to continually negotiate and renegotiate their religious identities, in ways that enable consonance between their religion and sexual identities. But these personalized forms of religion did not develop overnight. Many of the interview respondents in this study "shopped" for churches[6] in the period between their departure from the church in which they were raised and their arrival at Unity Fellowship Church. During their trial periods at different congregations, the respondents did not find what they were seeking; hence, they visited other churches. In this period of church shopping, however, emerging were increasingly personalized forms of religion. For most of the respondents, Unity Fellowship Church served as the turning point in their religious discovery. By this time, however, some of the respondents already possessed an undeveloped form of personalized religion, but it was the influence of Unity Fellowship Church that activated this religious form.

Interviews again and again highlighted how congregation members responded to the meaning of their religious identity, in relation to their sexual identity. The respondents tended to personalize their religious identity, adjusting it to some key areas of their life—notably, to their sexual identity. Certain self-feelings and psychic reactions were prominent in this personalizing process. For instance, individuals' verbalized feeling conflicted between their religious identity and their sexual orientation. Some of the respondents experienced confusion, fear, shock, guilt, and shame, while others became angry, in response to hearing homophobic sermons. They felt increasingly alienated from their former religious institutions, and experienced a diminished sense of worthiness as a result.

Yet, despite the animosity that many religious groups exhibit toward GLBT men and women, and in spite of the dissonance many gay and lesbian Christians experience between their two conflicting identities, many gay and lesbian Christians feel very strongly about both their religious beliefs and about their homosexual identity. Their feelings for each identity are so strong that they refuse to give up, or reject, either one.[7] How, then, does one harmonize these competing identities? The interview data suggest that it is partly through a restudying—here, by entering an alternative religious setting—that a person is able to make sense of the "true" meaning of religion and gain a new understanding about how one's sexual orientation is, in fact, compatible with traditional religious meanings. The integration of religion and sexual identity, however, seems to require a very individualized and personalized form of religion.

PERSONALIZED RELIGION: SELF-DEFINING RELIGION

The pathway to finding a personal religious niche, in both the organizational sense and personal sense, does not necessarily follow a linear path. Kambo, for instance, explored various faith traditions and, at one point, even felt as if he "needed to create my own religion," for neither traditional religion nor alternative religions were meeting his spiritual needs. He described his faith journey as follows:

I started looking at Eastern religion, 'cause I was feeling a whole thing about mysticism and stuff like that. So I started seeing things about sophism, about Islam, about Buddhism, about Taoism, about. . . . I just wanted to read about it, because . . . I guess I felt like I needed to create my own religion. Because what I was taught and what I was brought up on wasn't working, but I knew there was something. I just didn't know how to put it into words. I didn't have anyone to tell me. And so, anytime I got a book or could find some information about something else, it was like, "Okay." And I think I had read a book about the Broadway play *A Chorus Line*, and a couple of them people who were involved in that became Buddhists and they were gay. I was like, "Okay, maybe it's accepted there [in Buddhism]," you know. So I started reading about Buddhism, you know. And so, it really became about. . . . But I couldn't get away from the tradition of being in church . . . in the traditional black church.

PL: Because you grew up in it.

Kambo: Yeah, and I didn't want to lose that. I was like, Why do I have to give that up? I shouldn't have to give that up.

PL: It's part of you.

Kambo: You know, and so when I found. . . . 'Cause I had gone to Metropolitan Community Church, and it was good. It was nice, but it was like, "Hmmm." It's just not the same sort of thing for me.

Although Kambo did not need to create his own religion after all,[8] his religious journey highlights how religion has become much more individualistic, tailored for each person.

The respondents in this study defined "personalized religion" in two ways. First, they had specific criteria and expectations of what organized religion should entail. This includes: the ability to be openly homosexual; different religious perspectives and different worship styles; a sense of comfort; spiritual fulfillment; personal relevance; and the continuing need for black religious traditions. Second, for congregation members at Unity Fellowship Church, "personalized religion" also means: individualized scriptural interpretations and the ability to question scriptures and sermons; the ability to draw from other faith traditions; and a level of autonomy from the Bible and from congregational lessons.

PERSONALIZED RELIGION: CRITERIA FOR
RELIGIOUS ORGANIZATIONS

Andrew Yip[9] maintained that it is overly simplistic to assume that non-heterosexual Christians are inclined to leave institutional Christianity simply because of a lack of affirmation and acceptance. He felt that there might be space within a religious institution for GLBT worshippers to negotiate with religious authority structures on doctrinal and practical matters. Yip further noted that while many GLBT Christians *do* distance themselves from churches, many also choose to remain in the potentially stigmatizing environment and persist in their spiritual journey.[10]

Congregation members at Unity Fellowship Church, however, exited their prior congregations for one reason or another. Yet, most of the respondents stated that, in spite of their departures, they remained grounded in their religious tradition. Minister Pepper, for instance, indicated that she "turned away from the [Baptist] church because I didn't understand it." But she added, "Just because I wasn't going every Sunday or [participated] in the church didn't mean that I didn't learn, you know, from the foundation that God is available. In my mind, I knew that."

Organized religion for GLBT African-American men and women must contain various elements that, for the most part, are lacking in contemporary religious organizations and in contemporary forms of religion. The criteria for modern religious organizations must affirm congregants wholly.

Affirming Congregants' Sexual Identities
and the Need to Be Openly Gay

Samuel, who attended a COGIC, AME, and Apostolic church, realized that he could not stay in a traditional church, "[b]ecause of the rhetoric and the dogma." He insisted that he refused to support churches, financially or otherwise, that were not going to support him in his time of need, or that did not support his same-sex partnerings. Samuel noted that he has been long estranged from the traditional church because "I need to be someplace where I can be okay there with the message that I'm hearing . . . sits well with me. And I'm not supporting anything that doesn't support me." In other words, for Samuel, his relationship with his church must be mutually respectful and mutually beneficial.

Jackie explained that the Holiness church in which she was raised had so many proscriptions that:

> [B]y the time you were twelve, you had so many "no's" that you became the hypocrite, because you're going to try to sneak and tell a lie to go to the movie house, because that was not allowed. . . . But the time I was

fouteen or fifteen, I was a rebel. So I started hanging out with people that was like me in New York City. So I found out that they were a lot of little gay folks that lived up the street, and my mother and me lived on 118th and 8th Avenue, so we had to pass this gay bar every day. So Mom and them would make fun, and that would make us curious.

PL: It's like reverse psychology.

Jackie: Uh huh [yes]. So it became a joy and free thing. So when I left [the] Holiness [church], I went to the spiritual church, and they was the ones who started telling me Jesus loves me just as you are.

Jackie stressed the need for "joy" and "freedom" in her religious life. For Jackie, being "free" meant being true to oneself and not having to be ashamed of, or apologize for, one's sexual orientation. Being "free" in the institutional-religious sense, however, required a congregation that would affirm, or at least would not denigrate, people's social identities.

Kambo ultimately joined Unity Fellowship Church out of a need to look for a "new way of understanding God. . . . That was my most basic thing." He added, "I definitely wanted to be affirmed. I didn't want to be a hypocrite anymore." He went on to explain how he used to attend an annual gospel music conference, in which gay and lesbian people were very much prominent. When the AIDS epidemic hit the United States, however, people he saw at one conference became noticeably absent at the next conference, or conference attendees' health quickly deteriorated from one year to another. AIDS killed many in the gospel music industry, but according to Kambo, the epidemic also made many people go back into the closet, "trying to get away from homosexuality," or "just trying to pray it out and doing what we called 'being delivered from it.'"

But Kambo also would hear cases in which men went "on the down low," presenting themselves as heterosexual, but engaging in homosexual relations during the week of the gospel music conference, an event that Kambo described as the one week in the year that closeted individuals, including closeted married ministers, "get to be gay." Kambo, however, became wary of concealing his sexual orientation. He explained, "I didn't want to be a hypocrite. It got to the point where I didn't want to be a hypocrite anymore." For Kambo, thus, an authentic religion and authentic church allowed gay people to be openly homosexual. He found this in Unity Fellowship Church.

Shelly came from a Pentecostal church in which homophobic messages were disseminated from the pulpit with regularity. She described struggling with her sexual orientation and her religious need for years. Well into her adulthood, she finally decided:

[H]eck with it. I searched around for various places, trying to find some kind of refuge or some kind of safeness. So I believe that I was some freak of nature, and that I was doomed for hell. So I basically lived my life that way.

PL: Because that's what the church was telling you.

S: Yeah. I basically lived my life that way. I was on drugs and an alcohol[ic]. Prostitution. I did everything. I just got far away from that thing called church, you know? And, you know, 'cause I felt like I was going to hell anyways. So that's why I dissociated myself with the church.

The need to be openly homosexual (or even bisexual) in their respective congregations was a common theme among the interview respondents. While not all of the respondents were members of, or attended, congregations that were either overtly homophobic or that were, at the least, unsupportive of same-sex relationships, it was the respondents' belief that being true to oneself, and being honest to others, meant being able to openly disclose one's sexual orientation.

The Religious Connection: The Sensory Perception of Congregational Compatibility, Comfort, Home, and Love

Joy grew up in the Baptist church but has visited various mainline African-American denominations, including an African Methodist Episcopal (A.M.E.) church. She left the Baptist church, but it was not because she was unhappy with the church. Rather, she desired something more in terms of the sermon content. As she explained:

> At that time, I wasn't even thinking whether [the Baptist churches] were gay friendly. I just didn't like the message all the time that they preached. I kind of wanted to learn more. In most Southern Baptist types of churches, it's just a lot of preaching and hollering, and, you know, you kind of just get tired of that. With Unity, I kind of wanted to. . . . The difference, I felt, was Unity taught a little bit more. And from a different perspective. From being a lesbian and being gay. In a regular church, they don't. . . . If they address it, it's in a negative way, and who wants to hear that all the time?

Once again, a congregation member has underscored the need for a "certain kind of message" and a "different perspective," but this often translated to mean "gay-affirming."

Jarvis was raised in a Holiness (Pentecostal) church and his parents were religiously strict disciplinarians. When Jarvis left home for college, his church attendance ceased altogether. It was not until he met his current partner eleven years ago did he renew his religious commitments, but he did so at a church that was unlike the one in which he was raised. As Jarvis described it, he only decided to attend the Unitarian church because "It ain't like church. They don't be doing all this 'Amen' and 'Yeah, yeah, yeah,' and they don't talk about God." While he found something appealing about the Unitarian church, the novelty wore off quickly, and both he and his partner sensed something "missing" from the Unitarian church. As Jarvis explained it, the sermons at the Unitarian church became too lengthy and lecture-like. He and his partner became bored, and his partner, therefore, went searching for another church for the two.

Felicity referred to "feeling a connection" at Unity, but this connection translated to having a radical perspective on religion. As she explained it:

> [T]he other churches that I went to even after I got out here, I go once or twice and that was it. I could tell usually with the sermon, where the preacher was coming from and, you know. And if I wasn't feeling it, 'cause I felt it the first time at Unity. I KNEW. I felt that connection. I knew right then this is something for me. 'Cause even the way he talked about Jesus being a liberator. See, nobody ever talked about . . . just gave me that portrait of Jesus before. Jesus as a liberator and a rebel? Oh, yeah, I can get ready for that nicely. That does not scare me, see? And I guess it would scare a lot of other people, but that appealed to me . . . to the rebel in me . . . I guess that was what that was. So, I felt that connection that first time.

Samuel indicated he ultimately joined Unity because "I'm a truth-seeker. And I like to get to the truth of things. I was able to find the truth at Unity." Minister Macon ultimately joined Unity because of "the message." As he put it, "The message was one of freeing. It was not discriminating, and so I attended and eventually joined." Minister Macon's statement suggests that personalized religion, for congregation members at Unity, cannot be oppressive.

For other respondents, their need was more general; they simply needed to *feel* like they belonged to the church community. This was the case for Felicity, Gavin, and Candy, who "bounced around" from church to church before arriving at Unity Fellowship Church. The three respondents described feeling an immediate "connection" with Unity. Felicity explained that she could usually gauge her degree of comfort and connection with the first sermon. She stated, "I could tell usually with the sermon, where the preacher was coming from and, you know. And if I wasn't feeling it, 'cause I felt it the first time at Unity. I KNEW. I felt that connection." Candy added, "[At] some of the other churches . . . I didn't feel not welcome, but I didn't feel welcome. . . . When I first got to Unity, I felt like this is where I need to be. It just had the right feeling. It felt like home."

For the interview respondents, the "right feeling" often translated to the messages of love in the sermons. According to Joy, "[My first visit to Unity

Fellowship Church] was comfortable and it was just so much love in the [sermon] message. That was really the first thing, so it was just so much positive love in the first message." Selma concurred, but she relied more on a language that stressed equal rights and justice when describing her criteria for organized religion. She explained, "Everybody should be able to feel comfortable. If I pay my tithes and I pay my taxes, I have a right to come to my household of faith and be comfortable." For Selma, religion must exemplify man's humanity and love for fellow man. This, she stated, is the basis of her joining Unity Fellowship Church:

> I felt love when I needed a hug or needed to be loved. I'm telling you, people, when you come to church for the first time, you're coming because you're broken. And then when you get here and you hear the sermon and people was praying for you and stuff, and whatever you're going through is gone for that moment. I mean I felt comfort. My spirit, my soul, could rest.

Kaelyn described comfort in terms of congregational size. She has visited a local A.M.E. church. While she "felt the dynamics, the diaspora of the African-American community," she felt this particular congregation had an artificial feel to it. This was partly due to the size of the congregation, which lent an impersonal feel to both the service and fellowship. Kaelyn also described this congregation as having a "television kind of feel to it. . . . [I]t just felt . . . cathedral to me. And I was not comfortable." She went on to describe how the congregation had "big productions," "big screens," and a "huge" choir. In other words, the resources at this church were plentiful and prominent, in stark contrast to the no-frills appearance, resources, and approach at Unity Fellowship Church.[11] The grandeur of the large A.M.E. congregation she visited, however, contributed to what Kaelyn felt was a "rehearsed feel, as opposed to a natural flow of service."

These narratives highlight the need for congregation members to feel a sense of belonging, a sense of comfort, and a sense of community at their congregations. All of these elements, which are primarily sensory-based, were basic to what the respondents seem to characterize as a truly "authentic" congregation. Making a congregation one's home church required having a "right feeling" when one steps into the congregation, and experiencing genuine camaraderie and familyhood.

"Comfort" and a "sense of belonging" on occasions were highly specific. Kaelyn, for instance, demanded a congregational size that allowed for direct and sustained interactions between the ministers and the parishioners, and among the parishioners. The sheer size of the megachurch did not permit these close relationships and, hence, lacked the sense of community that Kaelyn desired. Among Candy's congregational criteria included a welcoming congregational environment in which members and visitors alike are unthreatened. She described how some churches will single out people and make people feel embarrassed and ashamed if they do not tithe $100 or more. For a church to "feel right," however—at least for Candy—the congregation must be genuinely inclusive of all people, and refrain from singling out or shaming people.

The Need to Be Spiritually Fed

While some of the respondent narratives revealed instances of homophobia and other forms of ideological oppression within religious institutions, not all the respondents in the study described a religious history filled with oppression. Rodriguez and Ouellette, in fact, noted that the desire to merge together one's homosexual and religious identities does not necessarily follow a period of identity conflict between the two. [12] This was the case for Minister Salihah, who grew up in the Catholic Church. Minister Salihah noted that he was "lucky" in that his Catholic Church pastor never preached homophobic rituals, laws, doctrines, or dogma, something he did witness while visiting a friend's church. Minister Salihah eventually left the Catholic Church, however, "not because of my orientation" but because he felt spiritually unfulfilled and "needed to transcend the whole Catholic idea of and really get a deeper sense for me. A deeper sense, a connection to God." In other words, he needed a religion and a theology that spoke to him intrinsically.

Similarly, Jones emphasized the need to be "fed" spiritually. He explained, "When I find what works, I don't stray. . . . I'm not looking to go to these other churches to find out what they have to offer, because I'm being fed right then and there." Yet he indicated that during a period at Unity Fellowship Church, when Archbishop Bean was touring the network of daughter churches, he was not being spiritually fed by the replacement pastor. As a result, he exited Unity until Archbishop Bean returned. He explained that during Archbishop Bean's absence from the church, "I just left. . . . I wasn't feelin' it. I mean, I wasn't feeling it. It didn't feel organic. It didn't connect with me spiritually. It didn't help me to achieve anything, so I just walked. I quietly left." [13]

Selma described what it meant to be "spiritually fed":

> You know how you're hungry and you eat something but you're still not full, you're not fulfilled yet? So it's like when you've been renewed and the whole nine yards, it's like you have had your meal, you're full, and you have your dessert, and it was complete. You are totally complete. It's like right now I'm complete. I feel . . . I don't know . . . I just . . . I still want to save the world, but I'm just motivated and rejuvenated. I can do whatever I want. And the more and more I learn and depend on God, then it gets better each and every day.

For Raymond, being "spiritually fed" meant:

Spiritually, I need to understand what's going on in the world. I need to understand what's going on in my life. I need to understand why is it that God loves for who I am, as being a homosexual man? Why does he love me? And why can't other people love me unconditionally like God does? And so, coming to Unity, I get that feeding. When the ministers are up there speaking about certain situations. . . . Because they don't just talk about what's in the Bible. They talk about life itself. What's going on in the world today. How certain things fit into your life. How certain things don't fit into your life or shouldn't be in your life. So it's not all about the Bible all the time at Unity. It's about what's going on in life today. That's what they speak about up there on the pulpit. They . . . they read from certain scriptures and things like that, to help you understand what they're talking about, so . . .

Minister Vicky noted that at some churches, messages, practices, and routines become so routinized and mechanical that one becomes bored and eventually feel as if they were no longer being spiritually fed. She explained that she grew up in a Baptist church, but that as a teenager she ventured out and began to explore other churches and denominations. She settled at a "spiritual church," but after the pastor died, she felt that she was not "being fed": "It was like just spinning wheels, just wasting my time going, because I wasn't feeling anything anymore."

Being spiritually fed has many meanings. For some congregation members, it means that their church is answering life's complex questions, doing so in ways that are understandable, in ways that make sense, and in ways that are personally relevant. It also means resolving life's many contradictions. For other congregation members, being spiritually fed means something else. It may mean that their church and the religious teachings it espouses are providing congregation members some form of positive energy, motivating them and perhaps even inspiring them to make a change for the better—whether that betterment is in their own lives through self-change or the betterment of other individuals and groups, through collective action.

A Comparison of Unity Fellowship Church and Local Gay-Affirming Congregations

Not all of the interview respondents had the opportunity to visit gay-affirming congregations prior to their arrival at Unity Fellowship Church. In fact, for some of the respondents, Unity Fellowship Church represents the first and only gay-affirming congregation they have attended. Candy, a life-long Baptist, admitted that she was not even aware that gay-affirming congregations, such as the Metropolitan Community Churches, existed.

A few of the respondents, however, previously had the opportunity to visit at least one gay-affirming congregation. As a college student, Kambo attended a gay-friendly, Afrocentric church in Washington, DC. Shelly and

Rhonda both attended a Metropolitan Community Church, although at different congregations. Kevin attended a gay Methodist church in West Hollywood, an experience that he succinctly described as "very nice," but "a little boring."

Kevin's partner, Antoine, visited a church that had gay members, but whose priest was only selectively out to members he knew to be gay. At first, Antoine indicated that this was a "gay Episcopal church," but then amended his description. He emphasized that this church was not a gay Episcopal church per se, but that he simply knew that the priest was gay and "He was gay to the members who were gay that knew he was gay, but he hid. He hid that. And he didn't ever preach on anything gay, even though there were so many gay members. And it almost like . . . he felt ashamed, a shame in that. . . . So to me it wasn't really a gay church." The selectively gay priest did not discuss gay-related issues from the pulpit. What struck Antoine as more odd still was that this priest also never preached about HIV, even though at the church there was a computer class for HIV-positive men.

A few of the respondents visited Agape Church, a congregation that Thomas[14] described as "metaphysical." Joy and Ramona both described Agape as gay-friendly, but not gay-centered. Ramona even insisted that Agape was not a "gay church," stressing that at Agape, the clergy never explicitly articulated the word "gay." She described the congregation as comprising "all kinds of people there," and even opined that "[i]t's more straight than ever." In fact, she felt that Agape Church did not "cater to the gay people. It's a facet of their existence." She pointed out that gay themes never really constituted the totality of Agape's church life, especially since when it was a heterosexual couple who ran that church.

The respondents' experiences at other gay-affirming congregations make it clear that as GLBT worshippers, their church needs to openly affirm GLBT identities and openly speak about GLBT issues. In other words, churches that were, in theory, gay-affirming could not simply sidestep the gay issue; to do so would mean that there was little difference between these so-called "gay-affirming congregations" and the more mainstream congregations that denied GLBT worshippers the right to be openly gay. For the respondents in this study, being *truly* gay-affirming meant that not only could people openly disclose their sexual identities at church, but that the preacher needed to discuss GLBT issues from the pulpit. In other words, a congregation cannot affirm a group of people while simultaneously suppressing the discussion of topics that affect that group and that matter to that group.

The Continuing Need for Black Religious Traditions

The interview data suggest that for some of the respondents, if not most, participation in a gay-affirming congregation was important. However, for

the respondents with deep religious roots, being gay-affirming was not suffi-
cient to make a church *their* church. It had to be rooted in African-American
religious traditions. The "authentic" church, thus, meant not only gay-affirming but Afrocentric; more specifically, it had to be grounded in black religious traditions.

Earlier in this chapter, Kambo described his exploration of various religious faiths, but he also explained how he "couldn't get away from the tradition of being in church . . . in the traditional black church." Similarly, although Samuel left "the traditional church" because it did not support him
during his time of need and condemned his sexual orientation, having been
churched all his life, there are religious elements that Samuel nevertheless
requires. As Samuel explained it, "See, for me I still need the basic elements
of what church is for me. Growing up in a Pentecostal movement, there are
just certain things that church has to have for me." These elements include
certain traditional church rituals and practices.

Shelly, too, could not get away from traditional church rituals, having
been in the COGIC church for so long. As she explained:

> I searched around. I searched around at different churches, but, see, that . . .
> that background, that belief was so ingrained in me that I couldn't find comfort
> nowhere, because I refused to be . . . the formalities of the COGIC. I was used
> to the holy spirit and singing and shouting and . . . you know, so I couldn't find
> comfort in these other places. It was not a comfort for me . . . until I came to
> Unity, and there a full gospel, you know, type of . . . whatever . . . your
> experience is.

Although Shelly has visited a gay-affirming congregation prior to joining
Unity Fellowship Church, she was not comfortable with that particular
church environment. She explained:

> I was not comfortable there. I was not comfortable there. See, because at this
> time, I knew the essence of myself was not gayness . . . that I was a person and
> had a soul and it was searching for salvation. It wasn't just about "we're all
> gay." You know, it was a little bit more to me than that. And I didn't want to
> throw out my total belief that I was raised in the fundamentalist of . . . Christ.
> The triumv . . . the father, the son, and the holy spirit. See, there was so many
> things I did believe, and these other churches didn't promote that. They didn't
> promote whole living. They didn't promote salvation. They didn't promote . . .
> I mean you pretty much just was gay and hallelujah and you can live and do
> anything you wanted. I still wanted to be a Christian. I still wanted to be
> "saved," you know?

Shelly went on to explain that because she came from "the old church," she
could not eliminate "the tradition." She felt that some of the gay-affirming
congregations, however, were "too gay" and that in these congregations, the

emphasis on sexual orientation and sexual expression meant an absence of moral lessons that "taught" people how to be "a good person, a good citizen, to not commit adultery, to not . . . lie, cheat, steal." For Shelly, gay-affirming congregations that stress the gay element primarily eliminated the moral element from religious services, as if homosexuality and morals (and social norms) were contradictory. But Shelly felt that gay people *could* be law-abiding, moral people. They could be "good Christians," and, most importantly, they could be "saved." Indeed, more than anything, Shelly wanted and needed to "be saved." She explained:

> During my years of drinking and abusing, I always wanted to be saved. I always wanted to be a child of God. . . . I thought—literally thought—that I would never have this because of my sexual preference. So I was very, very miserable. And I drank and used to try to make it go away, you know what I'm saying? So to be able to come home and to rest in his peace is having a little peace of heaven here on earth.

Thus, in spite of visiting several gay-affirming congregations, including a Metropolitan Community Church and an Agape Church, Shelly just did not feel comfortable at those churches. She felt that these churches overplayed the gay aspect and were insufficiently religious, in the traditional, ritualistic, and moral sense.

Ramona, who describes herself as "always been Baptist," dissociated herself from the Pentecostal church in which she was raised. This was around the time when AIDS was beginning to proliferate. She indicated that AIDS had tainted her views on religion, especially as a gay person, and so went out seeking her own church. But even after coming out and removing herself from her church, she described how God remained an integral part of her. She explained, "I always had God in my heart, [but] I never really sat down and decided on organized religion." She visited a Metropolitan Community Church, a non-denominational, gay-affirming congregation, but did not identify with what she described were "Catholic elements" at this particular church. She explained, "I know me and what I'm comfortable with." Going to a non-Protestant church, even if it were gay-affirming, however, was "not me. I don't force it . . . I'm not into that. It just wasn't me."

Here, Ramona underscored her need for a culturally affirming religious organization. She stressed, in particular, her need for black Baptist elements. Other respondents, too, stressed the need for an Afrocentric congregation. In other words, for some of the respondents, being gay-affirming was not enough; their church must reflect and affirm the congregants wholly, and that mean a racially-affirming congregation.

This was the case for Kaelyn, who grew up in Baptist and COGIC churches in the Midwest, and later became an "unofficial member" at a Metropolitan Community Church. She explained that the MCC she attended, which was a predominantly white church, did not provide racial or ethnic affirmation. She received the racial affirmation at Unity Fellowship Church, however. As she described it, when she first ascended the steps of Unity Fellowship Church, she felt "an instant connection, and I haven't gone back to the old church since. It was just . . . I think I entered in on prayer. Probably the African-American tradition roots, 'cause MCC is predominantly white, so it was just like an instant connection [at Unity]."

Kaelyn was ultimately drawn to Unity because of its roots in African-American religious traditions. This Afrocentric element instantly connected Kaelyn to Unity Fellowship Church, a connection that was absent with the MCC church. Indeed, she indicated that she left the MCC because she did not feel culturally affirmed, and that was in large part because the MCC churches are predominantly white. Kaelyn's experience suggests a need for worshippers to be affirmed wholly.

Samuel concurred with Kaelyn's sentiment. When I asked him what makes Unity Fellowship Church so special, he stated, "You cannot go anywhere, any other church in the city . . . that I'm aware of . . . especially not the black church movement . . . that are accepting of [gays and] transgenders. . . . In black traditional churches, that's not gonna happen." In other words, for congregation members such as Kaelyn and Samuel, it was important that their church not only be GLBT-affirming but Afrocentric. Black religious traditions must be prominent.

Unity Fellowship Church specializes in an Afrocentric, therapeutic form of worship. This is what some of the respondents had been missing. Archbishop Bean has constructed worship service as an emotionally and ideologically engaging experience that integrates the black religious and cultural traditions with GLBT issues. Unity Fellowship Church, thus, appeals to members because the church life is based on common cultural elements that are rooted in shared experiences as GLBT people, shared traumatic experiences, as well as a shared racial history.

While GLBT issues are prominent at Unity, there is much more to this church than affirming GLBT people. Unity is rooted in the black religious tradition, just as its congregants are. Archbishop Bean draws from the historical experiences of black Americans and from the rich traditions of black religion. Religious symbols are interpreted in ways that are relevant to congregation members, contextualized in this community's shared historical experiences. The religious rituals similarly are practiced in ways that respond to this community's social experiences.

At the same time, the respondents' continuing attachment to black religious traditions hints that some of the congregants are not necessarily gravitating toward excessively therapeutic forms of religion—or, in the Rieffian sense, "remissive" religion for purely self-interested reasons.[15] That is to say, while the respondents indicated a preference for a therapeutic form of religion, their continuing attachment to traditional black religion suggests a need for a structure that sets up rules and that guides and limits human behavior. Thus, the respondents' decision to become members of Unity Fellowship Church is not simply an excuse to focus on self-fulfillment and other psychological needs, or an excuse to behave in an unconstrained manner.

In summary, organized religion for GLBT African-American men and women must contain various elements that, for the most part, are lacking in both traditional and contemporary religious organizations and in both traditional and many contemporary forms of religion. The criteria for modern religious organizations must affirm congregants wholly. They cannot simply prioritize one social status at the expense of another, as evidently is the case with many of the predominantly white, gay-affirming congregations. They must also retain cultural traditions, while at the same time allowing more expansive ways to interpret and practice religion without alienating certain people or groups. Unity Fellowship Church represents a new form of organized religion, and a new form of religion, that contains all of these elements.

PERSONALIZED RELIGION: INDIVIDUALIZED UNDERSTANDINGS OF RELIGION

At the institutional level, the interview respondents outlined various criteria they set for religious organizations. They, too, also had very clear ideas about religion at the individual level. While the respondents understood that there was no single or uniform way of interpreting and understanding religion, they all believed flexibility was crucial for a religion that speaks to all people. This flexibility included at least three elements: the need to be able to question scriptures and sermons; the ability to draw from other faith traditions; and a level of autonomy from the Bible and congregational instructions.

The Need to Be Able to Question Scriptures and Sermons

For Felicity, the need to question the Bible is a crucial part of her form of religion. According to Felicity, believers need to be able to question scriptures and sermons, even if it goes against the church grain. In fact, she explained that the reason why she left the church[16] was the strict conformity required; she was taught never to question the Bible or to ask questions. Similarly, she knew she was not allowed to interpret Scripture for herself. Felicity further noted that before coming to Unity, "I couldn't find a place that allows me to think, because the churches that I was exposed to—and I dare say the ones that are still around—don't want you to think. They just want you to walk in lock-step. And I don't walk in lock-step with anybody."

Felicity expanded on her need to be able to think autonomously, without being bound by religion or her pastor's religious instructions.

> So the things that [Archbishop Bean] talks about from the pulpit. The things he's telling you: "You read. You interpret. You analyze. You question. You discover." These ministers don't want you to do that. . . . They want you to walk in lock-step with whatever their program is. And their program comes out of standard. . . . You know. You're a soc [sociology] major. You know the standard curriculum in colleges and universities that you follow to get your bachelor's, to get your master's, to get your PhD. You know. And you know there are standard doctrinaire kind of theory that goes along with whatever your major is. If you're outside of the box with that, you gonna have a hard time gettin' your degree. Now you know that, because your professors are gonna be looking at you askance and sayin', "Oh, she is a boat rocker."

Just as formal education seems to require that students conform to an indoctrinated way of thinking, analyzing, and writing, so, too, are congregants—students of religion—socialized to think in set or standard ways. Felicity attributes this trend to the formal educational system, which includes the religious seminaries, in which pedagogy is taught "within the box." Because Archbishop Bean was not schooled through formal channels, it is Felicity's belief that Archbishop Bean allows his congregation to think outside the box. This is because Archbishop Bean himself thinks outside the box. As Felicity described him, Archbishop Bean is a:

> Risk taker. He's out of the box. His sermons are going to be out of the box. His teachings gonna be out of the box. And most people don't do that. They don't. . . . Because then you got a congregation you can't control. You got a bunch of people who might want to take over. See, that's the way most people think. Oh, I can't liberate them. I can't set them free, because then they'll take over and where will I be? How will I be able to control them? See, but that is not, you know. . . . And I think a lot of ministers go into it because they go into it as a career path, not as a calling.

For Felicity, congregations and other formal institutions socialize people to think in one way, a practice that she believes is intentional, as it operates as a form of social control. It is Felicity's belief that if people were allowed to think outside of the box, they become uncontrollable, because that is when they begin to question authority. But for Felicity, it is crucial that she be able to reason on her own, and to reach her own conclusions and judgments on her own, without other people imposing on her their viewpoints.

In other instances, congregation members simply desired theological clarification, but their requests were dismissed or ignored. This was the case for Minister Pepper, who expressed how no one would help clarify Scripture or sermons when things "didn't add up." She felt the need to question religion at times, and sought religious guidance. One thing she wanted to understand was the difference between Jesus and God. But, as Minister Pepper put it, "[N]obody would tell me. No one would. . . . No one wanted to admit that there was a difference in the Baptist tradition. No one. . . . Either they didn't know or they didn't want to admit that there was . . . that there do be a difference."

Unlike Felicity, Minister Pepper was not actively rebelling against the established social order. Rather, she wanted the church to clarify ideas and, hopefully, resolve certain contradictions and misunderstandings. This process of clarification, however, necessarily involved questioning both the religious text and the religious teachings generated from the pulpit.

The Ability to Draw from Other Faith Traditions

For some of the respondents, personalized religion enables believers to draw from religious traditions outside of Christianity; in other words, they are not restricted to simply Christian beliefs and traditions. This appeared to be particularly important for Kambo, who described experiencing enlightenment from the Muslim tradition, as well as from Buddhist principles. He admitted, though, that he did draw from the Bible occasionally, "for strength." Other times, Kambo picked up non-Christian sources of inspiration and enlightenment, "because that's what I need at that moment." He felt this practice was acceptable, but wanted to assure me that he was not turning his back on Christianity when he relied on non-Christian spiritual resources.

Here, we see that personalized forms of religion expand the boundaries of possibilities, to include traditions and lessons outside of one's own religious affiliation. Kambo, thus, practices a personalized form of religion that draws from multicultural sources. But he was only able to do so because of the lessons he learned from Archbishop Bean, who often preached that God is "greater than any religion, denomination, or school of thought." According to Kambo, "[A]ll those things about me hearing that God was bigger than Christianity helped my spirituality." That is to say, the lessons learned at Unity Fellowship Church allowed Kambo to understand that he is not confined to simply a single religion on which to make sense of the world. At Unity Fellowship Church, the depiction of God as "greater than any religion, denomination, or school of thought" means that religious and spiritual inspiration can be found anywhere, even in unlikely spaces and places, and even in other religious traditions.

Safiyah visits other faith traditions, including a Jewish congregation during the High Holy Days, as well as a congregation that serves African immigrants.[17] In fact, Safiyah credits Archbishop Bean for peaking her interest in Judaism. She described her entry into Judaism:

[At] this job that I had for nine years, the president at the time was a female, and I came to understand that she was Jewish. And I was quite enmeshed in my liberation theology, but much credit to Archbishop, he always would explain the Judaic things that Jesus did. He never hid Jesus' Jewish background . . . like you find in some Christian churches. They are LOATH to even mention it. So they try to get as far away as that as possible. But not Archbishop Bean. And that started to really peak my interest.

Safiyah explained that she had plenty of questions with respect to Judaism, including: "What does it mean to be Jewish?" Why are Jews so hated? What have they done that they are so persecuted throughout history?" Moreover, she "really wanted to know who Jesus was." She elaborated:

Well, I knew who he is, but I wanted to know what it meant to be Jewish, because Archbishop always reminded us that [Jesus] is not a Christian; he's a Jew. . . . And so, those things really made me begin to question a lot about Christianity and then realize that clearly his [Jesus'] teachings are not Christian; his teachings are Jewish. He's coming from a Jewish perspective. And that made me want to know, well, what does it mean to be Jewish?

At one point in our conversation, Safiyah even referred to her "Jewishness." This occurred when I inquired whether she ever questioned any of the content of the sermons at Unity. She replied:

Oh, I don't know. I think it depends. I don't know. Probably, knowing me. I probably . . . I might question some things because that's my Jewishness. That's what Jews do. They go from Genesis to whatever, and they question every single thing, and they expound upon it and debate it.

PL: So you do consider yourself Jewish? At one point, early in the interview, you said "Christian."

Safiyah: You know what? I consider myself a Judeo-Christian. That's what I am. Because I would never let go of Jesus.

Personalized religion for Safiyah, thus, includes not only the ability to self-identify as something other than Christian, but also the ability to identify as having more than one religious identity concurrently.

A Level of Autonomy from the Bible and from Congregational Lessons

Finally, a few respondents suggested that personalized religion meant having a degree of independence from religion. Gavin best exemplifies this perspective when he noted, "You can't really depend on the Bible for all your daily life. You can't really. You can get inspired by it, but you can't depend on it. You know, you can get some inspirational words." For Gavin, more important than the Bible is one's ability to demonstrate the *essence* of God and biblical teachings—that is, to demonstrate love, even if in a non-religious manner. In Gavin's own words: "When it comes to the bottom line, it's everything is love. L-O-V-E. And that's the bottom line. I don't care what you read in the Bible. It's all about love. If you got love, and you can love everybody, I think you got it all licked. You got it licked."

Baylyn also pointed out that while she is sometimes inspired by the Bible, her sources of inspiration and personal revelations "might not come from the pulpit." In fact, her inspirational sources may not be religious whatsoever. Revelations, instead, may occur simply through "my own personal relationship with God."

NOTES

1. Swidler, *Talk of Love*.
2. Ann Swidler, "Culture in Action: Symbols and Strategies," *American Sociological Review* 51, no. 2 (1986): 273–86.
3. Swidler, *Talk of Love*, 93–94.
4. Ibid., 103.
5. Ibid., 93.
6. Sargeant, *Seeker Churches*, 41.
7. Rodriguez and Ouellette, "Gay and Lesbian Christians," 345.
8. Unlike Sheila Larsen, a respondent in Bellah et al.'s *Habits of the Heart*, who named a religion ("Sheila-ism") after herself.
9. Andrew K.T. Yip, "The Persistence of Faith Among Nonheterosexual Christians: Evidence for the Neosecularization Thesis of Religious Transformation," *Journal for the Scientific Study of Religion* 41, no. 2 (2002): 199–212.
10. Ibid., 201.
11. Funding and resource differences between the congregations are apparent.
12. Rodriguez and Ouellette, "Gay and Lesbian Christians," 346.
13. Congregation members have noted to me that Jones has since left Unity. I estimate his departure from Unity Fellowship Church sometime in 2006 or late 2005.
14. I did not interview "Thomas," but merely interacted with him informally at the church.
15. Rieff, *Triumph of the Therapeutic*.
16. Felicity attended Methodist, AME, and Baptist churches. She also attended a religious science church.
17. Safiyah is sponsoring a family from Africa, who attends this African congregation.

Chapter Four

Reconciling Religious Contradictions

The sexual orientation of many congregation members at Unity Fellowship Church represented a challenge to religion, and forced a new direction in the congregation members' religious and personal lives. But what happened when congregation members recognized that their homosexuality caused a clash in meaning with the teachings of the church? How did congregation members reconcile the contradictions? As Dawne Moon observed, and as I also observed, it was difficult, if not impossible, for congregation members to believe things in the Bible that went against what they knew about God and life—or at least what they *hoped* they knew about God and life. Interpretations of scriptures *had* to make sense.[1]

The data from this study reveal that congregation members undergo an identity reconstitution. This is a process they learn and develop at Unity Fellowship Church that enables a reconciliation of their GLBT and religious identities. The culture at Unity allows members to rework their identities and envision a gay life that incorporates religion, and one that views members as contributors to the community.

Certain religious-biographical patterns and orientations helped congregation members integrate their religious identities with their sexual (and other stigmatized) identities. These patterns and orientations include: the selective use of scriptures and sermons; understanding the context of the Bible; recognizing the Bible as man-made; using God as a theological rationale; self-direction; and application of liberation theology principles. Regardless of form, each strategy appears to be a highly individualistic, personalized way of understanding religion. Yet, they also draw on cultural resources—the assumptions, practices, and repertoires of their congregation. At times, congregation members use different strategies, depending on their situation, context, and needs. In some cases, congregation members utilize more than one strategy simultaneously.

INDIVIDUAL STRATEGIES

Sifting: Selective Use of Scriptures and Sermons

Lynn Resnick Dufour explored how women who identified as both Jewish and feminist created unconflicted Jewish feminist identities. By "sifting" through their available options, the Jewish feminists were able to construct fairly stable biographical identities that incorporated aspects of two or more potentially conflicting identities. They did so by cognitively, emotionally, and behaviorally selecting only certain attitudes and practices of their various reference groups, and then "trying on" or testing various attitudes and practices to see if they meshed well with their existing sense of the self.[2] This process of sifting, Dufour concluded, leads one to accept or adopt various practices and attitudes that "fall into" one's identity.

Because one uses different criteria to sift, the practices and attitudes that pass into one's identity may not all fit easily into one's life. One may identify with various practices, for example, that cannot all be enacted at the same time. To meet all of one's needs, Dufour maintained, one may have to selectively identify with a variety of reference groups, identifying only with select aspects of particular reference groups, and sifting out (i.e., ignoring or just not identifying with) the offensive aspects of the same groups.[3]

In the case of integrating one's sexual identity and religious identity, religious GLBT men and women may need to sift out certain religious teachings that reject their sexual identity, while accepting other aspects of the same religion that affirm their beliefs and statuses or that are otherwise personally relevant for them. This was the case for Shelly, who opined, "[T]he Bible is a good book and there are many good books. And each good book the author has its opinion. So, you know, you kind of take what apply and if it doesn't apply, you let it fly." The problem, however, is that people do take what they can use from the Bible to oppress others, a point that Shelly and other congregation members acknowledged. Shelly stated, "[T]he Bible can be very oppressive, but it's also very uplifting in its correct context [context]. See, we can make the Bible say anything we want it to say."

But are there certain elements from the Bible that we ought to sift out, or does it simply depend on the individual and on personal preference? Antoine seemed to have the solution:

> I'm going to tell you something that's really occurred to me . . . is being a writer and reading the Bible? The way it's written you can tell the person—some of these passages are written . . . [by] people with very high imagina-

tions, being that I have one. So you know that even though a lot of what['s] in that Bible, a lot of it is good. It does good, but then there's scriptures. . . . That's why I said go through the Scripture to find the good. Find the good. If it's something that makes somebody feel less of a person, and you know that by sharing that with them, that's going to destroy them. Leave that part of the Bible alone.

I don't think God is going to sit there and judge you on whether or not you believed everything that was in your Bible. But I do think he's going to judge you on if you killed your next-door neighbor. If you went over and fought people in a senseless war, when you knew . . . in a place in your heart that that was wrong to do. If you used greed to guide your actions. All these things that we do, we do. This is what God is going to judge us on.

For Antoine, it was necessary to "find the good" and sift out elements that make people "feel less of a person." He seemed partly motivated by his belief that God will, in fact, judge a person by his or her actions, particularly if there is a malicious intent behind said actions. Antoine's narrative, hence, not only illustrates one form of sifting, but it highlights how, in spite of being embedded in a religious culture that frames God as non-judgmental and always benign, Antoine continues to retain certain traditional images of God. Thus, partly motivated by a fear of a wrathful God, Antoine expressed his belief that people should retain only the "good" elements of the Bible, and omit the rest.[4]

It is not just the Bible through which congregation members sift. Although one might think that because the sermons at Unity Fellowship Church are affirming and inclusive, congregation members might fully embrace the sermons and not question them. However, this was not the case with the interview respondents. The respondents indicated that they, too, sifted through sermons, including Archbishop Bean's sermons. As Jackie explained:

[S]ometimes the sermon don't have nothing to do with what my thinkin' is. It's for someone else. And sometimes it's all for me. [I] look over some of the sermons that Bishop has preached that I didn't put with my story, my journey, but then I can find another thing he said . . . make it another moment that wasn't in the Thought for the Week. But that's what I needed.

Joy similarly admitted that she did not always agree with the sermons or the religious instructions, noting:

Every once in a while he'll [Archbishop Bean] say something, you know, I go, Okay. That doesn't seem right. . . . But the next person next to me might say, "Okay, that *does* seem right."

Ramona was more forthright as she explained:

> I have my beliefs and I have my ways of doing things. Maybe some ways are expressed in a way that a different clergy would not agree with. But, everyone has their own opinion and everyone's free to believe what they want to believe. I take away what I need to. I don't take away the whole thing. I'm not brainwashed, you know what I mean? I still have an identity. I take what I need from it.

In this statement, Ramona admits to sifting through relevant sermons, but she justifies this practice by couching it in terms of her own autonomy and her ability to think freely and intelligently. But she also added that she really only reviews the "Thought for the Week," or the sermon note, if it is "something pertinent that I can relate to" and "if it touches me in a way that I can really relate to and it'll be, 'Wow.'"

Other respondents similarly sifted only sermons and messages that were relevant for them. When I asked Selma what messages about HIV and AIDS the clergy at Unity were putting forth from the pulpit, she admitted, "I tune them out sometime. Like I'm saying, if it don't fit me, don't pick it up." In this case, since Selma is at low risk for HIV, the HIV/AIDS-related messages are less relevant for her.

Wanda, a life-long member of an Apostolic church until her arrival at Unity, declared that she combined both old and new beliefs and traditions, exemplifying another variation of sifting:

> I also take with me all this new tradition stuff that I've learned from here [at Unity Fellowship Church]. I also take my old, original beliefs, and I don't let go of that. I refuse to let go of my traditional home roots of spirituality and Christianity and religion [at the Apostolic church], so [I continue to] hold onto a piece of that . . . to go with this new modern, new contemporary . . . uh . . . stuff. Because this is by taking the New Testament and the Old Testament. Some people would totally want you to disregard the Old Testament. Totally disregard everything that was ever there, and you can't do that either. There's some stuff valid, some stuff that you [need]. . . . And you need to be able to recycle and weed them out.

In some cases, the respondents believed that sifting constituted a "right." This was the case for Rose, who asserted that everyone has "a right to their opinion. And I have a right to pick and read what I feel is best for me." This is a radically individualistic response, and one not without problems. If Rose believes that she has a right to "pick and read" from the Bible what she feels is best for her, then others have this right as well. The problem then becomes this: Sifting can lead to a distortion of intentions and meanings. Jones explained, for instance, how readers of the Bible, both past and present, sift through passages they deemed relevant, but often take words and meanings out of context in order to justify oppression. He stated, for instance, that whites interpreted the word "master" in the Bible as "white master of black slaves," and concluded that God was instructing the black slaves to serve their white masters. If congregation members at Unity have a "right" to read the Bible as they deem fit, do their oppressors have a similar "right" to interpret Scripture in ways that benefit them, even if the meaning and interpretations oppress other people? Again, this evokes the same moral dilemma that Antoine presented above.

Minister Macon hinted that all people—both the oppressed and non-oppressed—sift. That is, they take from the Bible what they can use, and discard the rest. As Minister Macon summarized, "The truth is [that] no one takes the Bible literally; they take portions of the Bible literally to benefit themselves, in their personal journey. But no one on this planet takes the Bible literally. It's impossible to live." Similarly, congregation members at Unity Fellowship Church take portions of sermons and scriptures that they deem personally relevant, picking and choosing aspects that are most meaningful for them and disregarding or screening out the rest, including beliefs that do not meet their spiritual criteria.[5] Critics might easily dismiss these respondents as simply "cafeteria Christians," but by selectively choosing interpretations to authenticate their own convictions, Roof would argue that the congregation members in this study are active "meaning-making creatures,"[6] and sifting is a cultural repertoire on which they draw to make sense of sermons and scriptures.

Understanding the Context of Biblical Writings

Some of the respondents combined sifting with contextual strategies. This was the case for Kaelyn, who has incorporated one of Archbishop Bean's exegetical lessons when she considers "the source of how it [the Bible] was written and the time it was written." But she also alluded to sifting when she added, "And that's the only answer I can say now and forever, because of my right to discern from it." Sifting, here, is transformed into a "right"; it is not simply an option or a privilege.

Similarly, Jarvis' approach to scriptures has changed over time. Prior to his arrival at Unity Fellowship Church, Jarvis indicated that worshippers would "stay confused" if they encountered scriptures that "didn't make sense." However, he questioned some of the scriptures even prior to his entry into Unity, and was able to discern, as he read biblical passages, "This is now. This was then." In other words, he considered the context in which scriptures were written, and realized that what was intended back then may not have the same meaning as in the contemporary context. As a result, Jarvis "will take what I can apply, and what I don't I just throw away."

Echoing the lessons of Archbishop Bean, Samuel explained that his approach to scriptures is as follows: "I take it all in with a grain of salt, because we realize . . . that [biblical] books come from other books, and the information that has been changed and manipulated, and most of the Bible in and of itself is based upon oral translation . . . oral tradition." Understanding the context of when scriptures were written has enabled Samuel to discern oppressive biblical passages more carefully, and to understand that passages that appear anti-homosexual were not necessarily intended to be homophobic. In some cases, these passages might not have been addressing issues related to homosexuality at all.

Shelly explained that she, too, did not take a literal reading of the Bible. As many of the respondents in this study did, Shelly echoed one of Archbishop Bean's lessons and emphasized the context of the biblical writings. However, she distinguished between changes in lifestyles and technology over time versus changes in "the messages." Shelly believed that, in spite of the drastic changes between when the Bible was written and now, there was a timeliness of the spiritual messages; she felt that the spiritual messages contained in the Bible remained relevant even today, for the most part.

Minister Calvin, a life-long Baptist, was not aware that the Bible contained oral narratives passed down from generation to generation until he heard Archbishop Bean's sermons. Minister Calvin admitted that prior to coming to Unity Fellowship Church, he thought that people simply "sat down and wrote the Bible." But the "fact" that the Bible is based on oral translations that are transmitted intergenerationally suggested to Minister Calvin that many of the biblical tales and interpretations were distorted as they were passed on to the subsequent generations. He elaborated:

> You know, if you had ten people in a room and you whispered something in one person's ear, by the time it gets back around, it's changed. So, I think there's a lot of stories . . . [w]onderful stories in the Bible, but in terms of accuracy, I just can't believe that all the information is accurate. And I think there's a bias based on who was writing, and since the majority of the writers were men, it's slanted to the male persuasion.

Rhys Williams maintained that cultural resources are "contextual in the sense that one cannot simply exchange one symbol or ideology for another. They are not worth the same—that is, they do not carry the same political weight—in each situation."[7] As some of the respondents suggest, individuals' application and use of scriptures may be temporal- and/or context-specific. Yet, people continue to use religion differently. Some people, for instance, use scriptures (or religion) to maintain traditional structures or beliefs, or to maintain traditions in the sense of perpetuating history. Other people may use scriptures to break away from traditions and beliefs that are obsolete in the contemporary context.

The interview respondents believed there were plenty of "spiritual truths" in the Bible. At the same time, they also believed that literal biblical interpretations might keep certain people and groups in bondage. The respondents' narratives further suggest that, for the most part, congregation members at Unity Fellowship Church view the Bible as simply a collection of writings and no more.

Recognizing the Bible as Man-Made

A few respondents emphasized that the Bible is man-made, echoing one of Archbishop Bean's lessons. This is reflected in Gavin's analysis of one unspecified Scripture that has been interpreted as anti-homosexual:

> [With respect to the passage about] men laying with a man . . . it's not right. No, that don't necessarily mean that. It didn't say that. If you were to go and read on, that's one person's opinion in the Bible. That was one person's opinion who wrote that book. That one Bible . . . Because maybe he had a reason why, you know. But God didn't say that. God didn't say it. That's what the man who wrote that book said: that man shouldn't lay with a man, and woman shouldn't lay with a woman. So that's the reason why . . . I question the Bible even more so now than I did before.

While the respondents recognized the Bible as man-made, as opposed to divinely created, the respondents still found much spiritual value and truth in the Bible. By acknowledging the Bible as a man-made creation, however, the content of the Bible—notably, the oppressive passages—is transformed into a human construction and is therefore moved out of the realm of divine command. That is, because the Bible is perceived as man-made—written by humans—the implication is that it is not God who is commanding the oppression of individuals and groups, but it is people who are oppressing other people. This epiphany meant that the condemnation of homosexuality—once thought to be biblical "truth," could be rejected. [8] Moreover, not only was the Bible written by man, it was interpreted by man, "with their slant on it, with their take," as Jones pointed out.

God as a Theological Rationale

Most of the interview respondents in this study believed that God was a beneficent, loving God. Their previous congregations, however, told them otherwise. The way that God is framed at Unity Fellowship Church, however, meshed with the respondents' ideas of what God ought to be: He is an always-loving God who "does not make any mistakes."

Painting God as inerrant is strategic: It suggests to worshippers that God has made people in His image, which includes GLBT individuals. If God makes no mistakes, then homosexuality cannot be deviant; indeed, homosexuality is considered natural, as well as divinely inspired. The God depicted at

Unity Fellowship Church, thus, is the God that *allows* a consonance of sexual and religious identities.

Although many of the congregation members at Unity long suspected that God was a loving God, they needed to hear it from the pulpit first. Minister Calvin alluded to this point when he stated:

> If people really thought about. . . . I mean really thought about the way some of these scriptures were interpreted in the Bible, they would say, "That just couldn't be," because that's the way I was. I was, "This couldn't be." God would not be that mean. It just wouldn't be. And I had no way. . . . I didn't know how to explain it. I just knew it couldn't be correct.

The verbal affirmation of God as always kind, always loving, and always at the side of believers confirmed for a number of congregation members at Unity Fellowship Church that God, in fact, loves the homosexual just as He does the heterosexual. In this way, God becomes the theological rationale for accepting homosexual worshippers, and for giving permission to congregants to openly and proudly be gay. Homosexuality, thus, is seen as not only natural but God-given. The homosexual worshipper, thus, is holy, because he reflects God. This is a particularly potent idea, considering the legitimating power is only in the hands of the divine, God. By anchoring homosexuality in the divine realm, the religious identities of GLBT worshippers at Unity therefore are considered legitimate.

This process is consistent with what Michelle Wolkomir[9] found in her study of gay and ex-gay Christian men who challenged dominant Christian ideology by taking small parts of it from the sacred into the secular realm for alteration, while leaving the legitimating power of the divine realm intact. All in all, Wolkomir found that a process of revisionist ideological work was key to aligning the men's perspectives with their respective groups, either a gay Christian community or an ex-gay ministry. This appears to be the case for Unity Fellowship Church members as well.

In the end, while the Bible has caused much turmoil among GLBT worshippers, it is *knowing* that God is on the side of GLBT men and women that enables a consonance. This pattern is summed up by Antoine:

> I studied that Bible so much, to whereas now I think I've gotten . . . I think God has pretty much gave me what I need, and it seems to be evident, because what Archbishop preaches on? It's messages that have already been given to me. So it's like . . . I don't need it. . . . Because I think God was saying what was twisting me up so long was that Bible. And I had to finally realize that Bible has caused so much confusion and so much division in my life . . . to whereas if I stopped looking for God to be in that Bible and just realize that he's always here, and he's what motivates, he's what sends me out, he's what brings me home.

In other words, Archbishop Bean has enabled congregation members such as Antoine to see that God is *within* believers, regardless of their sexual orientation. Therefore, GLBT men and women, too, are Godly and holy and there is no conflict between their sexual orientation and religious identity.

For other congregation members, reconciling contradictions involves more than simply acknowledging that God loves the homosexual just as He loves the heterosexual. It means learning to love oneself. Samuel, who has been at Unity for ten years, illustrates this trend. As he described it, he has now developed an acceptance of himself, and this occurred through a new understanding of God:

> I made it to an understanding of now there's really no separation between me and God . . . that homosexuality is not something that separates us. And that's huge, because so many of us still think that. See, if you believe that the God you serve doesn't like you, what's the real message . . . that you're receiving that they're not worth anything.

A lifelong Baptist who has also visited gay-affirming congregations, Ramona indicated that she has surrendered herself to God, but that her development is still "a work in progress." As she explained, her biggest challenge was "to find me where I could learn how to love myself." She noted that her life has changed considerably, for the better, but that:

> [T]o get to this point [is a gradual process], because I'm constantly being thrown at situations where I'm challenged and my faith is challenged too. Because I put myself out there, and I just give it to God and I actually believe that he'll take care of it in his time.

However, her relationship with God has given Ramona a peace of mind. She noted, "I have peace of mind in my home, my life, my work. Whenever I'm in a relationship, I have it there too. When I don't have those things, I take care of them because I love me. I love God first, then I love me. So, I don't let anything get in the way of those two things." Moreover, she acknowledged that by placing God first in her life, "[T]hings just kind of work out. It's having faith. Things are going to be okay. So, I can leave things there and just go on with my life."

Ramona is what we might call a deferring believer, or an individual who has developed a strong religious/spiritual identity based on deference to God. Deferring believers allow God to help solve their problems; indeed, deferring believers tend to let God be in control of their lives.[10]

Jones also may be considered a deferring believer, but with a twist. Describing how whites interpreted the word "master" in the Bible to mean "white master of black slaves," and that God was instructing blacks to serve their white masters, Jones highlighted how Bible readers, both past and present, often take words and meanings in the Bible out of context, in order to justify oppression. He explained, as a biracial (black and white) gay man, "My only master is God, and that's the God within me. The God that resides in every cell of my being . . . whether it's in a neutron or an electron or whatever . . . but whatever God exist in my being, that's the master that I have to serve. The only master I have to serve." Here, Jones completely defers to God. God is his master, and Jones is to serve his master, his God, loyally.

Jones obviously is not designating himself as God. Rather, he is claiming that with God "within" him, he becomes the master of his own body and spirit, and only he, and not others, has control over him. Technically, Jones is deferring himself to God, but this deference has a therapeutic twist: With God "within" him, Jones possesses a sense of self-ownership, autonomy, and agency, and he has the ability to resist oppression by others.

Self-Directing Believers

Earlier, Selma asserted with respect to exegetical strategies, "You have to come up with your own concept." She emphasized the need to open one's mind and consider other perspectives when interpreting scriptures and sermons. But even more important, according to Selma, is that people think independently with respect to the religious messages that they hear and read. Nowhere is this more prominent when she discussed her approach to scriptural text and sermons:

> [N]o matter what, even when the Bishop [Archbishop Bean]—or whoever your pastor is—that's preaching the Word, if you don't understand and you don't believe what he says, it's up to you to go re-read it until you get a clear understanding of what it is. And you take that and you go with that.

The aim, according to Selma, is to "to take the Bible and you have to read it and you have to understand to help YOUR life move forward."

In this single passage, Selma emphasizd the need to consider who wrote the Bible and the timeframe of the writing. When she asserted, "If it don't work for you, don't read it," she is highlighting the strategy of sifting. Finally, she also underscored the importance of autonomous thinking when she recommended, "You have to come up with your own concept." Thus, various strategies are at play simultaneously, but the goal is the same: developing an autonomous self. These strategies are consistent with religious individualism, which emphasizes the "sovereign self" and personal fulfillment. With religious individualism, an individual constructs his/her own personal religious identity by pulling together elements from various repertoires,[11] and religion and the role of religion are open to interpretation. This appears to be the case for Selma, as it is with other congregation members at Unity Fellowship Church.

Applying Liberation Theology Principles

Some of the respondents applied liberation theology principles to scriptural interpretations. For respondents such as Selma, liberation theology included the ability to open one's mind and consider other ways of understanding biblical text. That necessarily meant that the Bible is open to interpretation, a point that Baylyn underscored. Although Baylyn acknowledged that the context of the Bible must be considered, she also felt:

> [I]it's all in the interpretation. For instance, one of the biggest ones I use is Ephesians and it says, "Go be happy, little slaves." Now, back in the 1800s, when the slaves . . . when slavery was here and the Caucasian man would read that to the black man, he wanted them to say, "Okay, you're my slave. You have to obey." But now in liberation, how I interpret that scripture is, "No matter what you're going through, you can find joy in it. But you don't have to be enslaved by it." But know that it attributed to your overall path. And you have to walk the path of who you are; otherwise you'll never know.

In other words, an application of liberation theology to the Bible necessarily meant that the interpretations and understandings of the religious text must be freeing to people; it must advance the well-being of humanity, and not shackle or impede any single group of people.

INTERROGATING THE STRATEGIES USED TO HARMONIZE COMPETING IDENTITIES

The Self as the Reference Point

Andrew Yip's[12] study highlighted the lack of influence and impact of religious authority structures on nonheterosexual Christian views of sexuality and spirituality. In the construction of respondents' identity and Christian faith, as well as the fashioning of Christian living, religious authority structures were considered the least significant factor. More significant was the respondents' employment of human reason and biblical understanding, within the framework of lived experiences. Hence, in Yip's study, it is the self, rather than religious authority structures, that steer respondents' journeys of spirituality and sexuality.

We see elements of this tendency among congregation members at Unity Fellowship Church. Notably, the interview respondents relied on the self and the strength of their personal experiences, which they considered to be far more salient and significant than traditional religious mandates and teachings. For some respondents, the reliance on the self stemmed from a lack of confidence in traditional church structures and traditional church authorities, whom they deemed as dis-affirming, condemnatory, and as festering hate and fear. These respondents actively rejected traditional religious authority. In addition, most of the respondents linked "truth" and "authority" to personal experiences. By linking the lived experience as "truth," the respondents' personal experiences therefore become authoritative and are transformed into salient sources of religious authority. The self therefore becomes the ultimate reference point for the respondents' religious faith and practice.

The current study, however, deviates from Yip's conclusion that non-heterosexual Christians' ability to integrate two conflicting identities demonstrated the lack of influence and impact of traditional religion and organized religion on their personal lives.[13] Some of the respondents in this study have not abandoned their traditional religious roots. Indeed, black religious traditions remained important to a number of respondents, and rather than completing abandoning traditional religion, they drew from traditional black religious elements, while simultaneously incorporating other cultural elements acquired at Unity Fellowship Church.

Fluid Language, Fluid Interpretations

Claire Mitchell suggested that people's theologies tend not to be fixed. In fact, people tend not to have fixed ways of looking at the world, including at religion. Moreover, theological aspects of religious identification also respond to social and political experiences,[14] as clearly is the case for the GLBT worshippers at Unity Fellowship Church. For Unity Fellowship Church members, however, the allowance of flexible and shifting theologies is enabled through fluid language and fluid interpretations, which then allow congregation members to move and adjust themselves and their interpretations of scriptures, as well as their interpretations of the world around them, without feeling conflicted. As Bellah et al. noted:

> If the self is to be free, it must also be fluid, moving easily from one social situation and role to another without trying to fit life into any one set of values and norms, even one's own. In fact, one's values are not really a single "system," since they vary from one social situation and relationship to the next.[15]

The fluid language is evident in the respondents' ability to question, critique, and deconstruct scriptures, and in their ability to interpret scriptures (and sermons) in ways that allow a "fit" with their personal circumstances. In all, Scripture, sermons, and religious concepts at Unity are open to interpretation, and may be tailored for each individual, depending on the individual's needs. This fluid nature of speech (and, hence, action) can be constructed and reconstructed, rendering meanings and values more fluid, dynamic, and situ-

ational.[16] This characteristic allows congregation members at Unity to negotiate religious authority structures and oppressive scriptures. In doing so, they
are able to more successfully integrate their sexual identities with their religious identities.

Personalized Religion as Based on Shared Cultural Understandings

The interview respondents' narratives reveal highly therapeutic and highly
individualized ways of understanding religion and the world around them.
This includes the ways in which they relate to certain cultural points (e.g.,
scriptures, God, sermons, and other religious concepts), and in how they
emphasize the self as the reference point. Religion and religiosity are both
personalized, incorporating personal biographies, storytelling, and identity
politics. These strategies help congregation members organize their experiences and helps them evaluate their realities. They provide resources for
constructing strategies of action.[17]

Yet, the way in which the respondents relate to these cultural reference
points and the world around them are not constructed from scratch; they are
cultural products. That is to say, the respondents' personalized forms of
religion are based on culturally specific ways of doing things.[18, 19] As Read
and Bartkowski noted, "Discourses are not discrete ideologies; rather, they
are culturally specific modes of understanding the world that intersect with
competing viewpoints."[20]

Centering the self as the voice of religious authority and emphasizing
personal experience over traditional religious mandates appear to be pivotal
to the religious culture at Unity Fellowship Church. This point became apparent in the interviews. The respondents often cited themselves as reference
points for their religious outlook, so much so that for some of the respondents, it was evident that this particular cultural practice has been so ingrained in them that it now requires little effort and self-consciousness;[21] the
self as the voice of authority has become a taken-for-granted assumption.

Yet, the respondents are not cultural dopes. The interviews provide evidence that religious culture or social identities are not simply produced from
"above," from the rhetoric of cultural elites, nor are they passive conformists
who embrace every word of Archbishop Bean unquestioningly. Al nicely
summarized how congregation members remained autonomous beings, in
spite of belonging to a similar culture:

> [Unity Fellowship Church] allows you to be an individual at the same time
> belonging to a group. You have your individual beliefs and you have . . . but
> you can come together and still become a group. You know, everyone may not
> agree with the concept of heaven and hell. Some people do. Some people
> believe there are certain things that you should do; some people think you
> don't. But you can still come together on agreements here and find something.

You may not like what Bishop has to say; you may like what Bishop has to say, but you're allowed to express that and to feel that and know that no one is going to tell you, "Oh, you can't feel this, and you shouldn't do this this way," and, you know. Everyone's like, "Okay. You feel that way, but this is how I see it."

In Paul Lichterman's study, "personalism" meant *shared* ways of speaking or acting that emphasized the personal self.[22] In other words, in spite of differences in life experiences, lifestyles, and beliefs and norms, the one thing members of Unity Fellowship Church have in common is that they share a personalized approach to religion; that is, they embrace an approach to religion that is individual-tailored, self-expressive, and experientially based. They also often incorporate therapy into their personalized religion, which helps translate their experiences into personal meanings and, presumably, into social actions.[23] Thus, while personalized religion appears very individualistic, it is a shared practice and a shared way of understanding at Unity Fellowship Church.

Tapping from Different Cultural Resources

Some of the respondents drew their interpretive schemes from both standard cultural dramas and their own experiences. In such cases, the respondents did not feel the need to separate the two.[24] This was the case for Shelly, a lesbian raised in a strict COGIC church that explicitly condemned homosexuality. Simultaneously, she was struggling with a history of alcohol abuse, drug use, prostitution, and, ultimately, HIV infection.

Shelly searched for churches after her departure from the COGIC church. She even attended a gay-affirming congregation, but did not find comfort there. She felt the gay-affirming congregation was simply about being gay, rather than about being religious. To her chagrin, this congregation did not promote salvation, which was what Shelly needed more than anything. At the same time, because the COGIC tradition and beliefs were so deeply ingrained in her, she thirsted for some of the COGIC elements. How, then, did Shelly reconcile a deeply ingrained religious history that condemned her sexual orientation with her desire to find salvation as a lesbian? As she explained in her own words, her understanding of religion became individualized, deviating from the institutionalized understandings of religion in the traditional COGIC sense:

I know a lot about the religion, because not only was I raised in it, but my mother and father were ministers in it, and we were taught—we lived and breathed—that religion, that denomination, and their beliefs. So I couldn't very well far stray from it, so I had to stay with the Bible. But I have to find my truth in it. So that's what I did. And, yes, I studied the oppressive scriptures all the time.

It was not until she arrived at Unity Fellowship Church did she find comfort at a religious organization. It is apparent that the lessons at Unity Fellowship Church have rubbed off on Shelly, as she now embraces, and practices, more individualized, as well as more therapeutic, understandings of religion. Yet, Shelly is not simply expressing the perspectives and values espoused at Unity. Rather, she draws from her life experiences as a lesbian, alcoholic, and prostitute, and retains ritualistic elements from the COGIC tradition—notably, the concept of salvation. But it is only when she tapped into the cultural resources she acquired at Unity was she able to harmonize her religious identity and sexual identity. As she put it, "I'm VERY liberated at Unity. And very much saved and sanctified and feeling with the holy ghost [laughs]."

Wendy Cadge and Lynn Davidman's study of the religious identities of first-generation immigrant Thai Buddhists and third-generation Jews found that ascription and achievement were not necessarily conceptually distinct or exclusive ways of constructing religious identities. Rather, the respondents in their study combined ideas of ascription and achievement in their narratives of religious identity;[25] they fell somewhere in the continuum between religious identity ascribed by birth and that achieved as a result of conscious choices they make (and practice) to enact their identities. That is to say, their respondents neither simply emphasized choice nor ascribed religious identities and traditions. Many of the respondents actually remained within the religious (and ethnic traditions) of their birth, but used a mixed language of ascription and choice related to practice to explain what their identities are, if they see them primarily as religious or ethnic identities, and how they came to see their identities this way.[26]

Shelly appears to exemplify the trend found in Cadge and Davidman's work.[27] She is deeply rooted in the COGIC tradition and has retained much of the COGIC elements—notably the rituals. However, her religious identity (and, more significantly, the integration of her sexual identity and religious identity) is also partly achieved through the lessons disseminated at Unity Fellowship Church. Particularly with the concept of salvation, she has combined both ascribed rituals (and concepts) and achieved religious ideologies that pertain to the ability for homosexuals to be "saved."

CONCLUSION: INTEGRATING IDENTITIES

As members of Unity Fellowship Church sought to integrate their religious and sexual identities, they have learned from their pastor new habits and practices and new ways of organizing their own lives that, when accustomed, may shape their action.[28] Ann Swidler terms this process "cultural retooling." With cultural retooling, people: cultivate a new sense of self; incorporate altered ways of feeling and judging experiences; integrate new styles, skills, and habits of action; and change perspectives with respect to the nature of the world. These processes enable individuals to "enact new ways of being in the world."[29]

Congregation members at Unity Fellowship Church constructed their own religion and religious identities by drawing from various repertoires.[30] Some borrowed from other faith traditions. Others drew from the cultural resources they acquired at Unity. Others combined cultural resources, even if only situationally. Most significant, congregation members drew heavily from their own life experiences. Indeed, their construction of a positive integrated identity primarily rested on their own lived experiences. This was how they reconciled their religious and sexual identities. In some cases, respondents reinterpreted Christian doctrines and principles in order to formulate a Christian ethic that was consonant with their sexual identities. They drew from Unity Fellowship Church teachings, but also from their own lived experiences. The respondents' personalized religion is predicated on *their own* interpretation of the Bible, and of religion in general, and bounded in the framework of their own experiences. They also employed human reason to interpret the Bible.

A personalized religion that was based on the experiential and the therapeutic enabled a greater sense of peace and calm in congregation members. It allowed them to reprioritize demands and boundaries and to create new obligations and commitments that focus on the self. This form of religion helped congregation members to realize that who they are as GLBT individuals are precisely who they are supposed to be. It allowed them to become independent from the oppressive facets of religion. In all, personalized religion allowed the GLBT members of Unity Fellowship Church to assert their self-autonomy through religion, and to shape their own lives on their own terms, rather than on terms imposed by others. It allowed congregation members to self-define religion in ways that were personally meaningful, relevant, and empowering.

Integrating religious and sexual identities certainly was not a linear process for most congregation members in this study. Indeed, the process of reconciliation proved to be long and winding, and some respondents are still struggling to reconcile their identities. In the end, rather than having a fixed religious identity (e.g., the religious affiliation of one's childhood religious upbringing), many congregation members continually negotiate and renegotiate their religious identities. Throughout this process, they draw from various repertoires to make sense of religion. But no matter what cultural resources they appropriate, congregation members adapt them to their own purposes.[31] Findings from this study, thus, are consistent with David

Yamane's[32, 33] and Andrew Yip's[34] neosecularization thesis of religious transformation, which suggests that a person's religious orientation has shifted from the institutional to the personal. In a postmodern American society that places great emphasis on individualism and self-fulfillment, the respondents in this study also demonstrate an internally or self-referential system of constructing Christian faith, identity, and practice.

NOTES

1. Moon, *God, Sex, and Politics*, 63.
2. Lynn Resnick Dufour, "Sifting through Tradition: The Creation of Jewish Feminist Identities," *Journal for the Scientific Study of Religion* 39, no. 1 (2000): 94.
3. Ibid., 95.
4. This, of course, evokes not only a problem with dichotomies (the "good" versus the "bad" elements of the Bible), but the moral dilemma that inquires, "What constitutes "good" and what constitutes 'bad?" and "Who is to judge what is good and what is bad?"
5. Dufour, "Sifting through Tradition," 104.
6. Wade Clark Roof, *Spiritual Marketplace: Baby Boomers and the Remaking of American Religion* (Princeton, NJ: Princeton University Press, 1999), 43.
7. Rhys H. Williams, "Constructing the Public Good: Social Movements and Cultural Resources," *Social Problems* 42, no. 1 (1995): 127.
8. Wolkomir, "Wrestling with the Angels of Meaning," 412.
9. Ibid.
10. C. Jeff Jacobson, Jr., Sara E. Luckhaupt, Sheli Delaney, and Joel Tsevat, "Religio-Biography, Coping, and Meaning-Making among Persons with HIV/AIDS," *Journal for the Scientific Study of Religion* 45, no. 1 (2006): 39–56.
11. Robert Wuthnow, *After Heaven: Spirituality in America Since the 1950s* (Berkeley, CA: University of California Press, 1998), 9–10.
12. Yip, "The Persistence of Faith Among Nonheterosexual Christians," 199–212
13. Ibid., 203–4.
14. Claire Mitchell, "Behind the Ethnic Marker: Religion and Social Identification in Northern Ireland," *Sociology of Religion* 66, no. 1 (2005): 17.
15. Bellah et al., *Habits of the Heart*, 77.
16. Robert Wuthnow, ed., *Vocabularies of Public Life: Empirical Essays in Symbolic Structure* (New York: Routledge, 1992), 1.
17. Swidler, "Culture in Action," 284.
18. Jen'Nan Ghazal Read and John P. Bartkowski, "To Veil or Not to Veil? A Case Study of Identity Negotiation among Muslim Women in Austin, Texas," *Gender and Society* 14, no. 3 (2000): 398.
19. Lichterman, *The Search for Political Community*, 23.
20. Read and Bartkowski, "To Veil or Not to Veil?," 398.
21. Swidler, *Talk of Love*, 25.
22. Lichterman, *The Search for Political Community*, 23.
23. Bellah et al., *Habits of the Heart*, 127.
24. Swidler, *Talk of Love*, 38–39.
25. Wendy Cadge and Lynn Davidman,"Ascription, Choice, and the Construction of Religious Identities in the Contemporary United States," *Journal for the Scientific Study of Religion* 45, no. 1 (2006): 24.
26. Ibid., 36.
27. Ibid., 23–28.
28. Swidler, *Talk of Love*, 99.
29. Ibid., 75.
30. Wuthnow, *After Heaven*, 9–10.

31. Swidler, *Talk of Love*, 17.
32. David Yamane, "A Sociologist Comments on Sommerville: The Whole Is Less Than the Sum of its Part, *Journal for the Scientific Study of Religion* 37, no. 2 (1998): 254–56.
33. David Yamane, "Secularization on Trial: In Defense of a Neo-Secularization Paradigm," *Journal for the Scientific Study of Religion* 36, no. 1 (1997): 109–22.
34. Yip, "The Persistence of Faith among Nonheterosexual Christians."

Chapter Five

The Unintended Consequences of Therapeutic Religion

Therapeutic religion strives to equip the emotionally wounded with psychological capital, through open self-expressions, affirmation of social differences, and the provision of other freedoms otherwise disallowed in mainline congregations. While the intent of therapeutic religion appears sincere and noble, the freedoms that therapeutic religion permits and even encourages may have unintended consequences. In the case of Unity Fellowship Church, the therapeutic ethic appears to have produced certain excesses inadvertently.

EXCESSIVE RELIGIOUS FREEDOM?

The Church as a Meat Market

According to the interview respondents, general society tends to assume that gay people are promiscuous. It therefore makes little difference to church outsiders that Unity Fellowship Church is even a church. The fact that Unity Fellowship Church's congregation is overwhelmingly GLBT makes it less a church, and more of a space for gay people to hook up. The respondents indicated that, most often, outsiders view their church simply as "*that* gay church." This has various implications. According to Samuel, referring to Unity Fellowship Church as "the gay church over there" implies that the person is not taking seriously the image of Unity as a "real church." Characterizing Unity Fellowship Church as "*that* gay church" suggests that Unity lacks legitimacy as a real church in the eyes of perceivers. It also suggests that Unity cannot possibly be spiritual; it is perceived as a Godless organization, where sexual activities are assumed to be prevalent in all aspects of the religious and organizational life. The respondents, in fact, remarked how church outsiders—particularly those from the more mainstream congregations—commonly assume that sexual activities are rampant on the church premises. Al even pointed out how the general gay population in the area tended to assume that "everyone sleeps with each other here." Raymond concurred, stating, "By being a quote unquote gay church, they think they're [visitors] in a pick-up joint." Felicity also felt that a lot of people equated Unity to a night club, a sex club, or even a cult, and they assumed sexual activities occur on Sunday mornings, even during worship service.

Yet, some of the respondents acknowledged that, in some ways, Unity Fellowship Church was a meat market. The interview respondents pointed out that cruising was visible, even during worship services. As Raymond described it,

> [I]f you look around, people are not . . . Some people are not really paying attention to what's going on at the pulpit; they're looking around the church. Especially if there's new people who will come in. They put like a radar on you.

Jarvis described the pick-up attempts in even greater detail, observing the frequent physical movement back and forth—the departure from and re-entry—into the sanctuary to the common areas, all during worship service.

Raymond was quick to point out that these hook-up attempts are not limited to Unity Fellowship Church, and that he has observed these same behaviors at other churches, including the traditional "heterosexual churches." Indeed, some of the interview respondents suggested to me that people, from a very young age, are socialized to believe that they can find their future spouses at church. The assumption is that churches are the best place to find suitable mates, presumably because, as church-goers, prospective mates will be spiritually grounded.

Yet, Raymond also admitted that hook-up attempts are more frequent at gay-centered churches than at mainstream, traditional churches. Part of the reason for this, he believed, has to do with the fact that gay people have difficulty separating church life from night club life. But for a church such as Unity Fellowship Church, the hook-up attempts may be more rampant, simply because of the demographic characteristics of the attendees. As Raymond explained it, "For one, a lot of people at Unity are lonely. And so, they're looking for that fix that's going to fix them for that moment right then and there." Here, Raymond resorted to a psychological explanation for members and visitors' hypersexual behavior. At the same time, he also found these activities to be rather sordid:

> Because, see, people come . . . Church is like a hospital, as Bishop always says. You come there to get healing. And for someone to walk up and want to

pick you up as a date at a church, that kind of like . . . To me, that kinda like . . . I don't know. It kind of makes me feel dirty. You know, if someone's trying to pick me up in church? You know, we can do this afterwards, but while we're in the sanctuary, pay attention to what's going on up here. You know, sometimes Bishop say, "You have to separate yourself when you come to church with your lover. You guys have to separate. 'Cause you're too busy there hugged up with each other and this and that. Separate. Sit apart from each other."

A facilitator of a support group housed at the church who is not a church member himself indicated that some of the men at Unity Fellowship Church are "problematic" in the sense that they are overly aggressive in their pursuits of him. He characterized Unity Fellowship Church as a "meat market," in which men, in particular, are always checking out each other and coming on to each other. The support group facilitated pointed out that a male in his support group even boldly asked him if he wanted to have sex. The facilitator also indicated that not only will some of the men at Unity make verbal propositions, but they may stare at him inappropriately, in explicitly sexual ways that make him uncomfortable.

The clergy themselves are quite aware of the cruising activities that occur during worship services, as these behaviors are alluded to in sermons. In addition to the cruising activities, the clergy point out in sermons how congregation members frequently inter-date and change romantic partners frequently. But these behaviors apparently are not limited to the lay church members; a few interview respondents disclosed to me, without any prompts whatsoever, the relationship status and sexual behaviors of certain clergy. Some of the respondents even provided the sordid details about whom the clergy dated, and how these relationships developed. Thus, it became evident to me that even the clergy were implicated in the "messiness." That is to say, even church members themselves viewed the clergy's deviations from conventional religious and congregational norms as indicative of a lack of sexual- and self-control.

These behaviors, however, are not specific to Unity Fellowship Church, or to any gay-centered congregation. The search for romantic partners, both long-term and short-term partners, occur in all religious settings, but what distinguishes Unity Fellowship Church from the "other" churches appear to be the visibility and blatantness**[AU Query 2]** of the behaviors.

Loose Rules

Some of the respondents described Unity Fellowship Church as having overly lax rules. On the one hand, although congregation members unanimously embraced the logic behind the church motto "God is Love and Love is for Everyone," more than a few church members believed that the church's seeming "come as you are" mentality was far too relaxed. A number of interview respondents noted, in particular, the overly informal attire that some congregants favored. Candy, for instance, observed that the chuch's "come as you are" policy has led some members to wear outfits "that probably wouldn't be allowed at other churches"—the too-short shorts and skirts, the too-tight bodices, and, in general, clothing that revealed too much skin. Samuel, too, felt some of the church attire was a bit over the top. He singled out a male-to-female transgender church member who favored wearing extremely tight and low-cut blouses, exposing her ample breasts. He assessed her attire as "extremely provocative" and "very distracting," and further assessed her dress choice as intentional, stating:

> They know exactly what they're doing. It's not something that's done by accident. They know exactly what they're doing. And, you know, I think someone needs to, you know, say, "When you're here, you need to cover up and dress appropriately. Do not wear something of that nature to your mother's church."

While it is hardly unusual for some church members to criticize others church members' attire, Unity Fellowship Church members' critiques of fellow congregants' attire are significant because they suggest that, in spite of embracing freedoms that are otherwise disallowed at the congregations from which they fled, church members at Unity nonetheless wish to maintain boundaries and rules that demarcate what is appropriate and what is not, particularly in the context of a sacred setting. This desire to retain boundaries and structure, coupled with the desire to retain black religious tradition, indicate that the congregants are not oriented toward remissive forms of religion necessarily. Indeed, the congregants appear to recognize that, in spite of the flexibility of the rules and the freedoms that reign at their church, Unity Fellowship Church is foremost a church, with many of the same rules and boundaries as other formal religious organizations. In other words, simply because Unity Fellowship Church's culture and religion are more flexible and fluid, and more therapeutically inclined, does not mean that congregants can behave in unrestrained ways.

Sex from the Pulpit

The language and messages put forth from the pulpit are, at times, quite graphic, particularly the messages about sexuality from Archbishop Bean, who can be quite forthright. Two sermons stand out in particular. In one sermon, Archbishop Bean preached, "If you think an orgasm is good, then you should think about God." He was implying that one's spiritual relationship transcends the feeling that one obtains with sexual orgasm, especially since the latter feeling is fleeting. At another worship service, Archbishop

Bean referred to Jesus' morning erections: "If he [Jesus] made it to [age] thirty-three, surely he had a hard-on in the morning. If he did not have a hard on, did not find someone attractive, then he was not tested like me, like us." Archbishop Bean's point was that if Jesus were a real person, then he had to have had sexual feelings, just as most men do, and just as congregation members at Unity Fellowship Church do. Jesus, thus, is portrayed as flesh and blood. He is portrayed as a normal man, who was tested like the congregation members, and who faced trials and tribulations just as the congregation members did. He is a man, with the same feelings, the same temptations, the same everything that the congregation members possessed and experienced.

At first glance, the bedroom metaphors appear extremely explicit, perhaps too graphic for a sacred setting. When I interviewed congregation members, however, no one condemned Archbishop Bean's explicit use of sexual language, at least not for the above two aforementioned sermons. I observed that both above sermons were met with laughter, suggesting that congregation members did not feel that the explicit language was out of place or inappropriate; indeed, church members likely believed that the language was consistent with Archbishop Bean's style: blunt and humorous.

Nonetheless, most of the interview respondents, while understanding the humor of the sermon, did express some surprise at Archbishop Bean's occasional graphic language. A few respondents suggested that perhaps Archbishop Bean could have opted for a different choice in words. A few respondents, on the other hand, did feel that the graphic language was inappropriate for a religious setting.

Archbishop Bean's style actually is what is distinctive and important to his church community. He speaks in such an unrestrained, unvarnished way. He is not bound by what the Pope says, what other prominent black leaders say, nor is he bound by any denominational rules or religious tradition. He does not bite his tongue or beat around the bush, and he does not sugarcoat issues or sweep traditionally tabooed subjects under the religious rug. This style is agreeable to his congregants, and even gratifying. Congregants have expressed appreciation for Archbishop Bean's unreserved style, and they have described his messages as "real" and indicative of "truth." Shelly, for one, applauded Archbishop Bean's candor, stating, "That's why I love the Bishop. Because he'll say anything. He ain't got no shame in this game."

But Bean's blunt style also is part of the therapeutic relationship. Roger Betsworth, professor of religion, describes the therapeutic relationship as "one in which there is deep emotional bonding, a closeness between persons, and an honesty of communication."[1] While all three characteristics are present at Unity Fellowship Church, it is the honesty of communication— particularly by Archbishop Bean—that appears to draw people into the folds of this church.

But Archbishop Bean does not incorporate traditionally tabooed subjects in his sermons, nor does he use graphic or street language, in order to titillate. Instead, he seems to believe that talk—and particularly *honest talk*—is therapeutic in itself. Talk lends itself to healing, by allowing people to uncloak secrets that have burdened them, but talking also may lend itself to behavioral modification. This is where Archbishop Bean begins to resemble Sigmund Freud. Freud believed that instincts and impulses can never completely be suppressed, just as Archbishop Bean also believes that instincts and impulses can never disappear, for they are parts of human nature. To this end, both Freud and Archbishop Bean are confident that it is far more beneficial for both the individual and for society to talk openly about our instinctual desires and impulses, rather than repress them. By talking about our desires and instincts, and even allowing some expressions of these desires and instincts (i.e., sexual expressions), both Freud and Archbishop Bean believe that we can control our desires and impulses far more readily than if we were to repress them entirely. Indeed, Freud and Archbishop Bean both believe that the prohibition of behaviors and desires that otherwise cannot be contained can only result in destruction, either to the individual or to society. Their alternative, thus, is this: Rather than fully containing desires and instincts, at the least we must be allowed to talk about them, if not allow some expressions of them. In this regard, talk (i.e., language) becomes the essential medium of consciousness, and it is the essential means of liberation.[2]

CULTURAL CONTRIBUTORS OF THE EXCESSES

There is empirical and anecdotal evidence to suggest that various elements of Unity Fellowship Church's congregational culture—notably its therapeutic ethic—encourage excess freedom, even if unintentionally. The cultural contributors of these excesses include: overly individualized understandings of theology; a therapeutic understanding of God; framing sin and sinning in suprapersonal terms; medicalizing members' behaviors; and an absence of a proscriptive language. All of these elements, jointly or independently, facilitate some of the perceived excesses.

An Individualized Twist on Liberation Theology

Unity Fellowship Church's theology stresses individual therapeutic interpretations of theology. This church's version of liberation theology most commonly emphasizes liberation theology's intent to free people from shame, but the church's theology also provides allowances for people to interpret Scripture as they see fit, without having other people's demands and expectations imposed upon them. Kaelyn's definition of liberation theology illustrates this trend:

> Liberation theology tells me to think for myself and that is okay to do [so]. I
> have a right to my interpretation period. Whatever it is that's being presented
> to me or whatever it is I may be searching for myself. I've been given the
> power to think freely, based upon how my life has taken its turn. . . . Doesn't
> have to be oppressive anymore. Doesn't have to be male-dominated anymore.
> Female-dominated. My interpretation is okay. That's what liberation theology
> is to me.

Other congregation members stressed the psychological dimension of liberation theology; it was their belief that liberation theology aimed to free
individuals from internal psychological distress that arose from oppressive
scriptures. The respondents most often couched their definition in terms of
being able to be openly gay. Rose, for instance, defined liberation theology
as: "[being] free to be who I am . . . without having to worry about what the
next person thinks." Rodney interpreted liberation theology as "being liberated and being okay with who I am and not being in the closet . . . and not
being ashamed of who I am and afraid to say who I am and what other people
think who I am."

Some of the respondents couched their understanding of liberation theology in rights and social justice language, but even then the individualistic and
therapeutic strands remained prominent. This was exemplified by Candy,
who, while framing her interpretation of liberation theology in terms of the
principles of equality, ultimately defined liberation theology as an "all-ac-
cepting, all-inclusive way of thinking." Similarly, Selma described liberation
theology in terms of freedom, adding, "I have a right to choose and believe
how I want to worship."

By stressing individual understandings of theology and individual recovery, Unity Fellowship Church's liberation theology prioritizes the individual,
rather than the collective. That is to say, while collective action via group
participation in the struggle against group exploitation and social injustice is
mentioned in sermons on a regular basis—particularly in Archbishop Bean's
sermons—the core of the sermons, and Unity Fellowship Church's theology,
nonetheless remains focused on individual worshippers who are recovering
from various forms of social marginalization, including homophobia, racism,
economic disenfranchisement, and the stigma attached to a positive HIV
serostatus. In other words, the focus is on the self, and on psychological
recovery primarily, rather than a group participation in the struggle against
exploitation and social injustice. Given the congregational characteristics, the
individualized understanding of theology, however, is understandable if not
necessary.

A Therapeutic Understanding of God

Acknowledging their congregants' histories, the clergy at Unity Fellowship Church rely on a "vocabulary of suffering" or a "vocabulary of pain." The repertoire for relief from the pain is therefore a therapeutic God—a benign and loving God. Accordingly, at this congregation God is portrayed as steadfast. He is a caretaker, comforter, companion, decision-maker, leader, guide, teacher, parent, father, liberator, life saver, healer, deliverer, and savior. God is said to always be at one's side. God fixes messes, is in control, intervenes on our behalf, keeps people alive, liberates, saves people, uplifts us, validates us, and provides for us. Above all, God is said to be always at the side of believers, and to love unconditionally, in spite of congregation members' transgressions. Indeed, God is most often equated with unconditional love, or simply "Love," a finding consistent with Wilcox's[3] study of gay-affirming religion.

The messages at Unity Fellowship Church are clear: In spite of relationship fractures with family, friends, and others, God remains steadfast, always at the side of believers, regardless of their histories. In other words, God loves them, no matter what. Such a formulation of God is intentionally therapeutic. It fosters the perception that Unity members are cared for and esteemed.[4, 5] It suggests to congregation members and visitors that even if they are not loved by their (biological) families, they have another family here at Unity Fellowship Church and, always, they have a relationship with a loving God.

Such divine assurances and reassurances aim to instill in congregation members some semblance of hope, by mitigating sources of personal anxiety and distress.[6, 7] Yet, the therapeutic framing of God poses some challenges. For one, it invariably inverts the relationship between God and His believers, so that rather than believers serving God, God becomes a servant of His believers. That is to say, the clergy at Unity Fellowship Church focus mostly on what God can do for individuals, rather than what individuals can do for God. And even when congregation members praise and honor God, the expectation is that they will benefit from this action. Hence, it is not God who is at the center but the individuals themselves.

A second dilemma that stems from the inverted relationship is that the focus on congregation members' transgressions conveniently is eliminated. Because God's actions become the central point of attention, rather than believers' actions, congregation members are essentially freed from the responsibility associated with their transgressions. This point is made even more salient because God is said to make concessions on congregation members' behalf, particularly when they are lost and weak, and at their lowest point.

Given the histories and lived experiences of the congregation members, however, portraying God as angry, vengeful, as a despot, or in any other ways that downplay human liberty would be unsuitable. Many respondents described prior religious histories in congregations that put forth fire-and-brimstone sermons and provocative messages that depicted homosexuals as aberrant, abominations, and as destined for hell. These classical approaches to the divine are particularly hard to swallow in an age filled with catastrophic events, including the AIDS epidemic. In response, Archbishop Bean takes a psychological approach, by describing God in only upbeat, positive, and supportive terms, a strategy that is consistent with the therapeutic ethic.

Sin and Sinning as Suprapersonal

At Unity Fellowship Church, religion for the wounded involves a therapeutic understanding of the concepts of sin and sinning. Although sin and sinning are more often evaded topics, when the subject is broached in sermons, they are discussed in terms of social inequality and oppression; hence, the clergy frame sin/sinning not in individual terms, but in broader, structural terms. Such a framework is consistent with liberation theology, which often treats the concepts suprapersonally, or beyond the individual. Gustavo Gutierrez maintains that liberation theologians, in fact, often treat "sin" as not an individual, private, or interior matter, but as "a social, historical fact." By doing so, Gutierrez notes, "the collective dimensions of sin are rediscovered."[8, 9]

There is a conspicuous evasion of the concept of sinning at Unity Fellowship, at least as it relates to the biblical injunction against non-heterosexuality. However, based on what Archbishop Bean and the clergy say, as well as what they do *not* say, it is evident that nothing—not even egregious transgressions—disturbs or dishonors God. That is, the clergy never consider the possibility that the divine can suffer as a result of human sins, for God focuses only on divine joy.

Moreover, at Unity Fellowship Church, congregation members are seen as fundamentally good human beings, for the most part. As humans, of course, they are capable of transgressions, but these transgressions are usually not characterized as "evil" or "sinful"; rather, they are considered as simply "human." This point was highlighted when I asked Reverend Linda how Unity Fellowship Church addressed the concept of "sin" and "sinning." Reverend Linda explained:

> Well, our approach to sin is, really, sin is missing the mark. . . . So you've fallen short, you're failing, ok? You're not meeting the goal or the mark, and we all do that. We all miss the mark from time to time or in just different areas. So we teach more in that frame than from the "If you sin, then you're to burn in hell forever," removing that fear factor and that condemnation . . . .But we also present that God is a forgiving God, so even though we sin/miss the mark,

you are still worthy, and you can still be accepted in and grow in spirituality.
Or be accepted and loved by Christ.

Reverend Linda's statement reveals that the clergy at Unity Fellowship
Church have universalized the concept of sinning to *all people*. By universal-
izing sinning, sinning or "missing the mark" is normalized. Because "we all
do that," sinning is simply a mistake or human error. This dialogue also
reveals that Unity Fellowship Church views sinning as a forgivable act, and
that those who "miss the mark" remain worthy people.

It must be made clear that gay sex is not equated as "missing the mark,"
however. Same-sex sex is considered as natural as heterosexual sex, and as
"God-given." Reverend Linda's characterization of "missing the mark," thus,
really refers to acts that are unhealthy to the self and/or to others. This
includes promiscuity, relationship abuses, substance use, and criminal behaviors.

Reverend Linda also suggested that "missing the mark" represented congregation members' nonconformity to societal expectations, whatever those
may be. Thus, while members of Unity Fellowship Church do not consider
homosexuality as "missing the mark," larger society may interpret it as such,
and this is something Reverend Linda anticipated. Indeed, by applying
"missing the mark" to *all* people, Reverend Linda seemed to imply that even
if homosexuality were considered "missing the mark" (i.e., deviant), then
heterosexuality must be "missing the mark" as well.

My dialogue with Reverend Linda presents only one way in which the
clergy at Unity Fellowship Church frame the usually unspoken issue of sinning. An analysis of my field notes of worship services and sermons finds
alternative framings of "sinning" at this congregation. Usually, "sinning" is
never explicitly mentioned. Instead, it is referenced more subtly, couched in
secular language, rather than biblical ones. In addition, assessments of what
constitutes "evil" or "sinful" tend to center on behaviors and systems, rather
than on individual persons, and these acts tend to be described as oppressive
rather than evil, for the most part. That is, at Unity Fellowship Church, good
and evil do not simply reside within individuals, but are more reflective of
larger society, as social issues (i.e., racism, homophobia, and other forms of
social inequality).

And even if congregation members did commit a transgression, they are
not perceived as having sinned against God. If anything, their pastor believes
that they have sinned against themselves, by placing themselves in a perpetual state of torment and suffering through internalized hate and feelings of
guilt. But even if they did sin, either against God or against a fellow man,
Archbishop Bean insists that his congregation members are always governed
and protected by God, for a good and loving God would never abandon them.

In spite of the absence of an explicit language on sinning and, by extension, punishment, Archbishop Bean and the other clergy hope that congregation members will alter their behaviors. Indeed, the clergy seem to believe that congregation members can change their ways if they simply surrendered to God and "walk" with God. Archbishop Bean's sermons, in particular, often carry the implication that if people simply surrendered to God and maintained a genuinely inner or spiritual connection with God, they inevitably will discard their transgressive ways and live a spiritual, Godly life.

Even with good intent, framing sin and sinning as suprapersonal may contribute to the cultural excesses at this religious organization. By framing sin simply as simply "inequality" or "oppression," or as beyond the individual, the clergy at Unity Fellowship Church completely sidestep the individual, volitional aspect of sinning. Christian Smith, however, stated that an emphasis on the suprapersonal nature of sin does not negate the personal dimension of it. Gustavo Gutierrez also pointed out that unjust situations and conditions do not happen purely by chance, as "there is human responsibility behind it."[10, 11]

But there is a clear distinction. Smith and Gutierrez both focus exclusively on social injustice and the motivations and actions that lead to, and cause, large-scale harm to groups, populations, and even whole nations. The clergy at Unity Fellowship Church, in contrast, while they do underscore social justice issues, gloss over the volitional aspects of their congregants' transgressions. That is to say, by emphasizing large-scale injustices (e.g., inequality, racism, etc.) as sins, the clergy at Unity Fellowship Church divert attention away from small-scale sins: the individual-level behaviors and actions that cause harm to other individuals. In other words, attention is shifted away from personal infractions to larger social problems. The attention is then directed toward more abstract large-scale social problems, as they are more consequential to society as a whole, rendering personal, one-on-one infractions trivial in comparison.

While large-scale social problems such as racism and homophobia very well might have instigated certain individual acts of transgressions (for instance, drug and alcohol use and high-risk sexual behaviors)—and this causal relationship is often alluded to in sermons—missing from the puzzle is the volitional nature of some of the transgressions. To be sure, congregation members often operate under very constrained conditions, leading to a greater propensity to engage in high-risk and even illegal behaviors. Nonetheless, individual accountability cannot be subtracted from the equation.

Indeed, a few of the interview respondents felt that the sermons could emphasize more the role of personal accountability and personal responsibility. A review of my copious notes and transcripts from the sixty-one worship services I attended also revealed a noticeable absence of the theme of personal responsibility. However, when questioned, some of the clergy insisted that the sermons did, in fact, emphasize personality responsibility. As Minister Calvin explained:

> One of the big aspects of Unity and liberation theology is the concept of the devil. And Unity doesn't believe in the concept of the devil. That there is this person or thing that's making you do stuff. That's a cop out. You are doing stuff because you choose to do stuff. There is not a being making you do stuff. If you don't choose to do something, you don't have to do it. So instead of blaming it on the devil making you do it, be accountable for it. The devil is not making you smoke that cocaine, that crack pipe.

The Church as a Hospital

The clergy at Unity Fellowship Church on occasion equated their church to a hospital. This hospital metaphor was problematic in the eyes of some of the respondents, who felt that it allowed church members to sidestep over the volitional aspect of human behavior, allowing congregation members to pass on the responsibility for their own actions. Safiyah, for one, expressed her frustration when she stated:

> The first thing that gets on my nerve is that they refer to [this] church as a hospital, and I think that gets some of the cuckoo-for-Cocoa-Puffs people license to just act out any kind of way they want. So I'm not quite in agreement that that's a hospital. You know, it's a church . . . for spiritual enlightenment. And to learn how to love your neighbor, even as yourself . . .

Selma also felt that likening the church to a hospital had a deleterious effect on congregation members, in terms of their assumptions, attitudes, and behaviors. Like Safiyah, Selma felt that medicalizing or pathologizing congregation members' problems, and equating them as "patients," excuses their transgressive behaviors. Selma firmly stated:

> I'm still trying to deal with the fact that people say [Unity] is a hospital. No, this is church. You come here to get cleansed, to get help, to help you keep makin' it each and every week. This is not a place that you come and you bring your turmoil and your cheatin' and all that stuff. It's horrible. . . . [W]hen you come to church, a place where you worship, those are supposed to always be sacred ground. You should never bring unnecessary drama to the church.

That is to say, these respondents believed that the focus on congregation members' poor psychological states effectively evaded any personal responsibility. The blame is attributed not to the transgressor's own motives and volition, but to the conditions that "forced" them to engage in highly unconventional activities that they otherwise might not have engaged in had their lives not been so deprived.

Absence of a Proscriptive Language

Finally, at Unity there appears to be an absence of a proscriptive language. This absence, however, is consistent with the congregation members' backgrounds. Time and again, the respondents described histories at congregations in which their congregations and faith traditions communicated messages of "thou shalt nots," as well as condemnatory messages that denounced their sexual orientations. The language that characterizes Unity Fellowship Church's faith, however, is not a language of taboos and renunciations. At Unity, sermons stress "thou *can.*" Messages and lessons at Unity, thus, are not interdictory but instead give permission to congregation members and emphasize human potential and human possibilities. Understandably, Archbishop Bean and the clergy intentionally avoid a proscriptive language, because such a language necessarily implies restraint, restriction, prohibition, and social control of a population that has so little freedoms in their daily lives. Unfortunately, the absence of a proscriptive language may have unintended consequences, including unchecked behaviors among congregation members and the failure to take personal responsibility for one's actions and outcomes.

NOTES

1. Roger G. Betsworth, *Social Ethics: An Examination of American Moral Traditions* (Louisville, KY: Westminster/John Knox Press, 1990): 88–89.

2. Rieff, *Freud: The Mind of the Moralist*, 368.

3. Melissa M. Wilcox, "When Sheila's a Lesbian: Religious Individualism among Lesbian, Gay, Bisexual, and Transgender Christians," *Sociology of Religion* 63, no. 4 (2002): 497–513.

4. Ellen L. Idler, "Religious Involvement and the Health of the Elderly: Some Hypotheses and an Initial Test," *Social Forces* 66, no. 1 (1987): 228.

5. Anthony M. Pilla, "A Healing Progress," *Health Progress* (May–June 2001): 15–20.

6. Bryan Wilson, *Religion in Sociological Perspective* (Oxford: Oxford University Press, 1982).

7. Scott Schieman, Tetyana Pudrovska, Leonard I. Pearlin, and Christopher G. Ellison "The Sense of Divine Control and Psychological Distress: Variations Across Race and Socioeconomic Status," *Journal for the Scientific Study of Religion* 45, no. 4 (2006): 530–31.

8. Gustavo Gutierrez, *A Theology of Liberation* (Maryknoll, NY: Orbis Books, 1973), 175.

9. Smith, *The Emergence of Liberation Theology*, 35.

10. Gutierrez, *A Theology of Liberation*, 175.

11. Smith, *The Emergence of Liberation Theology*, 36.

Chapter Six

Therapeutic Religion and Ambivalence

The Case of Wanda

This chapter presents the case of Wanda. Wanda, a male-to-female transgender person, highlights some of the deep tensions and feelings of ambivalence that GLBT worshippers may experience when they are in an environment that not only affirms them but that provides allowances not acceptable at the religious organizations to which they were once deeply rooted. Wanda's ambivalence is most palpable in her critiques of aspects of Unity Fellowship Church's congregational culture, and of fellow church members. She expressed disappointment in what she perceived was the lack of personal growth among some of her fellow congregants. She described the church rules as overly lax and rarely enforced, and believed that congregation members were too lascivious and lewd on the church premises. She appeared to believe that some congregation members and church visitors used the church and its "liberal church teachings" as a license for sexual opportunism. Her assessment can be summed up as follows:

> Just because you're liberal over here and, you know, you've got the liberated theologian title over here, that [doesn't] mean that you can still sleep around with four or five different guys now. He's not going to accept that. . . . God is not going to bless a mess—whether it's a straight mess or gay mess. You know, bless a mess. So if you're having a partner over here and you're sneak[ing around]. . . . [If] it's not accepted over here in the heterosexual church, [then] it's not accepted here [at Unity] either, whether you're liberal or not. . . . [Just] because [Unity members are] saying we're liberated [theologians] . . . does not give you the license to still do all that other stuff. It doesn't. God expects wonderful things out of [gay people], just like He does with heterosexual people. He expects your loyalty, your commitment, just like it

91

over here. But to me it's just. . . . You know, here at Unity it's just a little too
liberal for me.

Wanda suggested that at Unity, there was "room for a lot of improve-
ment." One specific area that she felt needed change was in the church's
overall orientation. Specifically, she believed Unity "should be a little less
worldly, a little less carnal." Moreover, it was Wanda's opinion that Unity
needed "less allowing or making excuses." Again, she emphasized that simply because this particular congregation embraced liberation theology did not
give church members the license to form irresponsible interpersonal alliances
and engage in reckless or promiscuous behaviors. Nor should Unity "be a
hiding place for gay people, lesbians, and those with HIV. It should not be a
place where people can hide under the name of spirituality and Christianity."
Wanda underscored the church's need to insist to its members that they
cannot "half-step to salvation."

Acutely aware of the stigma attached to gay-affirming congregations,
Wanda was adamant that church members "walk in the light" and maintain a
consonance between religious instructions and actual behaviors. It was Wanda's belief that if church members exhibited high levels of personal and
social responsibility, in line with the teachings of Christ, gay-affirming
churches such as Unity would no longer be regarded as inauthentic, illegiti-
mate, or cultish, or as encouraging promiscuity. In summary, Wanda perceived her church as overly liberal, and she felt that the freedoms were far
too expansive at her church, leading to behaviors and orientations that are
otherwise not tolerated at the more mainstream, more traditional churches.

It should be noted that Wanda grew up in an evangelical, theologically
conservative denomination, and has attended only this one congregation all
her life before coming to Unity. The new cultural capacities that Wanda
learned at Unity likely incompletely altered her cultural repertoire, which
continues to include elements of her older cultural styles and strategies at-
tained at her former congregation.[1] This might partially explain Wanda's
rejection of what she felt was an overly lax style at Unity, and what she
perceived were loose morals of some of her fellow congregants. Yet, Wanda's dissatisfaction also hints to some of the limits of therapeutic-religious
societies, and draws attention to the ways in which therapy and fulfillment
can operate both as a source of pleasure for sexual liberation, but also a
source of conflict and constraint.

None of the other interview respondents detected the connection between
their church culture and congregants' (mis)behaviors. Indeed, most of the
respondents appeared very controlled in offering criticisms about their
church, and the critiques tended to be reserved for certain individuals and
individual behaviors. However, some of the respondents did subtly hint to
some of the church's excesses. This was particularly evident with respect to

their evaluations of the church's "come-as-you-are" mentality, which, in their eyes, permitted congregants and visitors to come to church in too-provocative attire, and to openly display overtly sexual behaviors.

On the other hand, Wanda was not alone in her ambivalence. One clergy acknowledged that some of the congregants were far too promiscuous. Despite what she viewed was the church's success in reaching out to marginalized members, this clergy opined, "I'd love to see people [at Unity] start thinking above the belt buckle." This statement suggests that not all the congregants have internalized the safe-sex messages and messages promoting interpersonal and social responsibility. But then, one would not expect that church members who come out of brokenness will change overnight. As one clergy described it, "It's a work in progress." Kyla, a congregant, added "[W]hen people come to Unity, they just don't suddenly become informed and empowered. It's all a process. So, you meet people on the different spectrum of the continuum. It's a continuum."

Most of my respondents—and notably the clergy respondents—denied that Unity's therapeutic ethic was problematic, hedonistic, or even overly self-focused. The typical response was that healing and self-focus were "necessary" to strengthen the individual before s/he can embark into mainstream society and live a healthy and productive life. Selma, however, was one of the few respondents who believed that therapeutic religion potentially could handicap congregants. Although she felt that some people needed "more nurturing" than others, she also felt that sometimes her church needed to simply let people help themselves. As she described it:

> I think at Unity sometime we handicap people, 'cause we don't hold them responsible for their actions. We want to sit up there and say, "It was their upbringing. It was mistake. They was molested as a kid and it's the anger that they went through as kid that. . . . " But I still believe that, regardless of you were brought up in a church or not, when you come to church, a place where you worship, those are supposed to always be sacred ground. You should never bring unnecessary drama to the church.

Wanda's reservations about therapeutic religion are understandable. Yet, one might wonder why Wanda does not simply change congregations, given her noticeable discomfort with this new form of religion. The answer appears to be this: It seems that Wanda does not—or cannot—leave Unity because the same elements that she critiques are ultimately the same elements she needs and desires. Wanda's ambivalence occurs because she is torn between two seemingly disparate religions and congregational cultures and has yet to find a way to merge elements of traditional religion with elements of contemporary religion satisfactorily, in a way that does not create dissonance between the two forms of religion.

In spite of her vocal critiques, Wanda had plenty of raves for Unity. In fact, although she was most vociferous in her critiques of Unity's congregational culture, her evaluation of Unity was positive, for the most part. She particularly credits Unity for its acceptance level, a point particularly salient for a transgender worshipper. As she noted:

> One thing I said I have to give Unity the credit, because they're most accepting. I mean I've seen people come to the doors that were completely drunk and irate . . . even spitting on people's faces in there. And they're very embracing. They're very embracing. You can be high as a balloon and you're not going to get knocked down. You know what I mean? You may have people that personally frowned down on you, but overall those doors will be open to you.
>
> People that are broken, that have been battered and scorned against—the minority, the ones—the ones that have been running away from all the other churches. They'll be comfortable there [at Unity]. You'll find that you're okay there. And that's a good thing. For those that have been beat up on and, you know, told that they can't. . . . People look at you because you don't have a nice outfit on and all dressed up, all sharp. You can come to Unity in your overalls and it's okay.

NOTES

1. Swidler, *Talk of Love*, 92.

Chapter Seven

Articulating Limits and Boundaries

The culture at Unity Fellowship Church in many ways represents the counter-culture to mainline church cultures. However, Paul Lichterman notes that the term "counter-culture" often is connoted as hedonism, degeneration, or generally a lack of commitment.[1] On occasions, the environment at Unity Fellowship Church appears to give the impression of hedonism, seemingly illustrating what Philip Rieff feared: modern culture's focus on remissive functions that free individuals from previously renunciatory control. Indeed, according to Rieff, modern culture has "shifted toward a predicate of impulse release, projecting controls unsteadily based upon an infinite variety of wants raised to the status of needs."[2]

The growth in remissive cultures aligns with the rise of therapeutic cultures in contemporary times. Among religious organizations, just as many theologically conservative Protestant cultures have shifted toward "psychological Christocentrism," Unity Fellowship Church also has gravitated toward the therapeutic. In this new orientation, congregations downplay suffering and sacrifice and emphasize and even promise happiness and fulfillment. James Davison Hunter summarizes that in these psychological religions:

> Subjectivism has displaced the traditional asceticism as the dominant attitude in theologically conservative Protestant culture. There is some variability, but in mainstream contemporary American Evangelicalism, an austere instrumentalism has been replaced by a malleable expressivity.[3]

Rieff was openly critical about the rise of the therapeutic, which he described as follows:

> [The therapeutic has arisen] out of a rejection of all therapies of commitment, precisely by persuading halfway the recalcitrant among those who submitted

to the old commitment therapies that they have acted out denials of knowledge and pleasure that no longer contribute to their spiritual health but, rather, to their mental dis-ease. So recently deconverted, the once-committed is unlikely to preach seriously against himself, except in terms of a historical drama, so that the therapeutic may enjoy his triumph.[4]

Congregation members at Unity Fellowship Church described feelings of alienation from their prior congregations, which denied their identities as GLBT people. The sermons at Unity are replete with descriptions of these prior religious histories, which tend to emphasize how these oppressive religions contributed to the mental "dis-ease" of congregation members. By instilling in congregation members fear and shame, some congregation members turned to underground activities, which only exacerbated their conditions of deprivation even more. Given these histories, it is not surprising that members of Unity Fellowship Church thrive in a culture that emphasizes individualized expressiveness and that allow liberties not otherwise present at traditional religious organizations.

But these freedoms are problematic, according to Rieff, because modern therapeutic culture seems to remove any sense of responsibility from individuals.[5] Therapeutic cultures, instead, emphasize gratification, impulse release, and unconstrained and unrestricted freedoms, and they fail to impose restrictive demands.[6] Modern "psychological man," Rieff argued, even aims to be free from "all divine suspicions."[7] This concern is one in which some of the interview respondents in this study observed as well. Some of the respondents, for instance, expressed concern about the lack of responsibility among some congregation members, whom they viewed as interpreting liberation theology far too loosely, in ways that suggest that this theological orientation allowed people to do as they pleased.

Yet, Rieff was aware of no culture that escaped the tension between the modalities of control and release. Rieff felt the tension between control and release existed in every culture and "even when the releases are devised cleverly (or dialectically) enough to allot to the controls of their superordinate function."[8] One might argue that this is the case with Unity Fellowship Church, where its release, in the form of "liberation" and human autonomy, may be said to be disguised in the guise of social justice, or in the language of rights.

Rieff likely would characterize Unity Fellowship Church as representing a "cultural revolution," in which the releasing or remissive functions and ideals become more compelling than the controlling ones. At that point, the tension between control and release reaches its breaking point. At that point, Rieff states, the culture

can no longer maintain itself as an established span of moral demands. Its jurisdiction contracts; it demands less, permits more. Bread and circuses be-

come confused with right and duty. Spectacle becomes a functional substitute
for sacrament. Massive regressions occur, with large sections of the population
returning to levels of destructive aggression historically accessible to it. [9]

Rieff further maintained that once the "releasing symbolic" exceeds the
controlling one, the culture is in jeopardy, because it can no longer support
the incumbent moral demands; rather, the remissive culture contradicts the
moral demands, even rejecting them. This signals the destruction of the culture, which cannot reconstitute its modalities of control, nor develop new
ones, because the modern remissive functions that characterize the culture
can no longer aggregate men for communal purposes, [10] instead intent on
satisfying the "erotic illusions" of individual men. A large part of the destruc-
tiveness of culture, according to Rieff, has to do with modern "psychological
man's" desire to be freed from institutional discipline and traditional morality. [11] Without institutional discipline and morality binding people together,
and without unity, a culture breaks down.

Rieff might very well have argued that, although cultures tend not to
escape the tension between the modalities of control and release, Unity Fellowship Church departs from his expectations in that it represents a very
distinct case in which no tension exists between release and control. That is
to say, to Rieff, Unity Fellowship Church would represent a culture in which
the ideas about, and the operatives of, release supercede those of control.
That Unity Fellowship Church is seen as a "meat market," that "loose" rules
organize congregational behavior, and that there are occasional graphic language from the pulpit all point to a culture that prioritizes release over control.

But the freedom that reigns at Unity Fellowship Church is not to say that
Unity is without order, morals, or control. To outsiders, the rituals and inter-
changes at Unity may have no order, but even this seemingly disorderliness
has order. The "disorderliness" is part of Unity's therapeutic style: It is part
of the free expressions and displays of emotion, affection, and styles, and it is
a celebration of differences. The high emotions, the flamboyance that characterizes some lifestyles, and the occasional heated interpersonal exchanges all
hint at an orderly disorderliness that characterizes a congregation that is
healing and, presumably, growing spiritually, personally, and collectively.

In some circumstances, the establishment of a repressive code might be
beneficent and even of social value. According to Freud, however, a repressive code is not beneficial in the therapeutic context. [12] Archbishop Bean
clearly embraces Freud's perspective in this regard, for he rejects repression,
particularly with respect to sexuality. But are there boundaries set for congregation members at Unity Fellowship Church, or does Archbishop Bean simply let freedom run unchecked?

Archbishop Bean is permissive, and he does not openly reject permissiveness. In fact, he embraces it. But this is not to say there are no boundaries at Archbishop Bean's church. Rieff[13] and other cultural scholars, however, likely would characterize Unity Fellowship Church as the ultimate remissive organization, but contrary to the seeming unrestrained expressions at Unity, there are limits to what congregation members can do, and should do, at Unity.

A therapeutic understanding of liberation theology among Unity Fellowship Church members appears to have led to a conflation of liberation theology with liberalized theology. According to cultural scholars, this may lead to a relaxed sense of duty, authority, and virtue, and a tendency to reject institutional religion itself, often on the grounds that it is morally hypocritical.[14] Certainly, critiques of both institutionalized religion and mainstream religious organizations are recurrent at Unity Fellowship Church, and there can be no doubt that the congregational culture that marks this church is a relaxed one. But the freedom that reigns at Unity is not to say that Unity is without order or boundaries. In fact, in sermons Archbishop Bean will articulate some of the boundaries with respect to what he deems is appropriate and what is not appropriate. In some ways, this goes against the grain of social control—the very same forms of social control to which congregation members rebelled against at their prior congregations. However, because Unity Fellowship Church is a church first and foremost, boundaries must be set.

Given the rampant stereotypes and misconceptions about his church, and of gay people in general, Archbishop Bean knows he must draw boundaries. This is particularly the case with sermons that discuss the sexual behaviors of GLBT people. Archbishop Bean cannot *not* talk about sex—granted that his congregation is GLBT—but he is also careful that he does not conflate homosexuality with purely sexual activity. The route Archbishop Bean takes is this: He grounds sex in religious terms—as Godly and, therefore, permissible and even divine. By doing so, he elevates his congregants—indeed, all gay people—to the realm of the divine.

At a religious class, and again during worship services, Archbishop Bean proclaimed that God was the vehicle for which humans expressed sexuality and suggested that incorporating God into one's sexual life represented a good health habit. Here, Archbishop Bean demarcated between healthy and unhealthy (sexual) relations by noting that healthy relationships were mutually respectful and therefore godly ones, while unhealthy relationships merely moved "from God to base lust and need." The message became clear: "Sex is not the same as love."

Here, Archbishop Bean argues against promiscuity in the following way: He suggests that sex without companionship cheapens the relationship, as there is no real companionship involved. The implication is that a purely physical relationship necessarily lacks substance because God is omitted from the picture. The act of intercourse itself—indeed, all intimate relationships generally—is framed in both psychological and spiritual terms. "Healthy sex" and "healthy relationships" are said to be based on genuine companionship, responsibility, and mutual respect, elements that are present when there is self-respect, which, presumably, occurs when one has integrated God into one's life. In contrast, purely physical/sexual relationships are grounded in carnal desires and are godless relationships. Sex coupled with companionship, thus, is permissible, because it is spiritual. And because it is divine, the act of intercourse, which includes same-sex intercourse, is therefore elevated into the realm of the divine.

While giving congregation members permission to express themselves openly, Archbishop Bean also is keenly aware of the stereotypes that surround GLBT people—that is, the perception of GLBT individuals as overly promiscuous. In response, Archbishop Bean regularly emphasizes the need to stop depicting gays, lesbians, bisexuals, and transgender individuals as simply sexual beings. In one sermon, he preaches the following:

> It's time for us to believe that we are more than sex machines. We are more than about sex. We are whole beings. We work, we are creative. It's time for them to stop thinking of us as sex machines.

He went on to state:

> [We must] challenge ourselves to see God and see the temple of God and not see body parts. We must see the whole person. In Christ, there is no male, female, transgendered, lesbian, gay. . . . [Y]ou need to identify yourself as more than [gay]. . . . You're a mother, a father. . . . It's not just about your sexual identity and who you have sex with.

Archbishop Bean's point here is that GLBT individuals are not simply sexual bodies. Rather, they are whole beings, capable of thinking and feeling and functioning in productive and gainful ways. They are creative beings, with multiple social roles and functions.

It is evident that Archbishop Bean has established some boundaries for his congregation. But the congregation members themselves *want* rules and boundaries. In fact, the respondents' perception of the loose structure and rules of their church, and their assessments of fellow congregants, suggest that, in spite of embracing some freedoms that are otherwise disallowed at the congregations from which they fled, church members at Unity Fellowship Church wish to maintain boundaries, rules, and traditions that contain excesses and that demarcate what is appropriate and what is not. Indeed, most, if not all, of the congregants continued to hold normative expectations of their church. This desire to retain boundaries and structure in the context of a sacred setting indicates that the congregants are not oriented toward purely remissive forms of religion necessarily. Indeed, the congregants appear to recognize that, in spite of the flexibility of the rules and the freedoms that reign at their church, Unity Fellowship Church is foremost a church, with many of the same rules and boundaries as other formal religious organizations. In other words, simply because Unity Fellowship Church's religion is more flexible, more fluid, and more therapeutically inclined than traditional religion does not mean that congregants can behave in unrestrained ways.

Conversely, while therapeutic societies may focus heavily on the individual, members of therapeutic societies do not think of themselves in purely psychological terms necessarily, nor are they exclusively self-indulgent. The interview respondents did not think of themselves in purely psychological terms, at least not consciously. To be sure, the prevailing therapeutic climate at their church has encouraged therapeutic understandings of the self. However, a number of respondents in this study, while recounting a history of sexual, physical, and emotional abuse, as well as experiences of institutional homophobia, at no time attributed their transgressions to these prior circumstances. This suggests that congregation members at Unity Fellowship Church are not simply blindly following their church leader and uncritically accepting certain therapeutic and cultural practices.

And contrary to claims that the therapeutic ethic merely fosters self-centeredness, the respondents in this study are civically engaged in their church community in one way or another. In fact, in spite of embracing concepts such as self-seeking, self-expressions, and self-love, many, if not most, of the respondents participated in activities for the communal good— for their church community, the larger community, or both. Participation ranged from cooking and selling church dinners to helping with other fundraising events, to participating in the church choir, to organizing the annual convocation in which the network of churches gather at the mother church, to helping with a literacy program, to participating in a literature and poetry event. One group even participated in a weekly street ministry, feeding and clothing the homeless every Friday night in the Skid Row section of downtown Los Angeles. Other congregation members participated in "smaller," quieter ways, engaging in the less visible, behind-the-scenes work.

These collective efforts suggest that, in spite of a distinctly therapeutic ethic that characterizes the congregation, congregation members at Unity Fellowship Church are not so inward-oriented or self-involved as to neglect the needs of others. Perhaps Lichterman[15] stated it best when he suggested that rather than judge a group according to communitarian models, which tend to be anti-individualistic and anti-therapy, it might be more appropriate to evaluate a group by the goals they have implicitly set for themselves.[16] Two of the most basic goals at Unity Fellowship Church include: 1) to provide a space to worship and fellowship together in ways that celebrate social differences; and 2) to provide a safe space for healing marginalized members.

Thus, while critics of therapeutic societies would describe Unity as too psychologically-oriented and insufficiently communal, the fact of the matter is that Archbishop Bean is not striving after a superior communal end, at least not in the immediacy. He cannot prioritize communal goals, given the more pressing needs of his congregation members, which include needs related to health and daily survival. Archbishop Bean also does not assume that a communal orientation is instantaneous, automatic, or naturally arises from church participation. His most basic goal is to offer marginalized and traumatized people unconditional love, along with a safe space to worship. In this respect, a truncated understanding of liberation theology—or, more broadly, the therapeutic ethic—may be more appropriate than a faithful interpretation of theology.

At Unity Fellowship Church, sexual identity and sexual expressions are not private matters. They are very public matters, and sexual expressions are openly encouraged. Some of the interview respondents in this study exhibited ambivalence to these trends, which are facilitated by the church's therapeutic ethic. On the one hand, the openness that the therapeutic ethic allows—has allowed—congregation members to heal. On the other hand, some of the allowances of this ethic have contributed to perceived excesses that appear to reinforce stereotypes of gay people. It also has led to skewed perceptions of this church by community outsiders, including the members of local, more mainstream and more traditional churches.

If outsiders disapprove of the practices associated with Unity Fellowship Church, as the interview respondents have articulated, it would seem as though the area for contestation is not that Unity Fellowship Church is a gay church per se. That is to say, it is not that members of the general public or that "other churches" disapprove of homosexuality but, rather, they may disapprove of the overt displays of sexual behaviors and sexual expressions. The ambivalence of some of the interview respondents also suggests that the tension is not about being openly gay; rather, the issue has to do with the spectacle of overt sexuality.

At Unity Fellowship Church, sexual individualism is emphasized, and pleasure from sex is lifted out from under the carpet. This has led to an unusually permissive, and sometimes sexually charged, environment in which certain acts and expressions that are seen to violate conventional religious institutional norms are rendered visible. This spectacle may suggest to both church outsiders and church insiders that the social order has broken down at Unity Fellowship Church. The visible behaviors at this church—the rampant cruising activities during worship service, the overt displays of sexuality, and the permissive language from the pulpit—are behaviors construed as going against the main purposes of religion, which include: regulation and restraint;[17] reinforcement of self-control; maintenance of moral standards; and, historically, the rejection of sexual individualism (which includes a divorcing of pleasure and procreation).[18]

The unorthodox displays of sexuality at Unity Fellowship Church, the blunt language of Archbishop Bean, and even what some might consider "inappropriate relationships" and "inappropriate behaviors" may all appear to be pathological by-products of a radically individualistic and radically therapeutic culture. But all of these things matter far less than the fact that the congregation itself is one that opens its doors to anyone and everyone. To church outsiders, excessive freedom characterizes Unity Fellowship Church, but to insiders this church represents some of the same freedoms that they, as African-American GLBT people, cannot possibly enjoy in mainline churches, or even in their life outside of church.

Moreover, the visibility of some of the observed excesses at Unity obscures the fact that the pastor has articulated limits and boundaries for congregation members, and that congregation members *desire* rules and boundaries. Findings from this study further indicate that although this therapeutic-religious society is anchored deeply in the personal realm, members are not simply using the community to enhance or enrich themselves. While there is a distinctively individualistic vocabulary and a prominent therapeutic thread in both the interview narratives and sermons, members of Unity Fellowship Church care deeply for their church and for fellow church members. This is indicated by their participation in various charitable church activities, however visible or small—actions that belie arguments that therapeutic societies necessarily are purely self-oriented, self-centered, narcissistic, and disengaged from communitarian goals. Thus, while therapeutic societies may focus heavily on the individual, members of therapeutic societies do not think of themselves in purely psychological terms necessarily, nor do they engage in only self-fulfilling activities.

Unity Fellowship Church is a vital religious community in which members share a world of suffering. This community is compassionate toward people with non-normative statuses and histories, because this religious community is a community with a shared history of human suffering. Thus, the imperfections of the church members matter far less than the fact that this church is a model for compassion. There is no doubt that therapeutic societies are not perfect. But this study suggests that there is something far deeper and of greater significance in the therapeutic cultural movements that characterize contemporary religion and society. Indeed, this case study maintains that a therapeutic ethic can actually serve important purposes for individuals, but the purposes, too, extend beyond the individual. Yet, it cannot be underscored enough that the therapeutic ethic is not a cure or end-all.

NOTES

1. Lichterman, *The Search for Political Community*, 255, footnote 20.
2. Rieff, *Triumph of the Therapeutic,* 17.
3. James Davison Hunter, *American Evangelicalism* (New Brunswick, NJ: Rutgers University Press, 1983), 91–101.
4. Rieff, *Triumph of the Therapeutic*, 254.
5. Ibid., 77.
6. Ibid., 254.
7. Ibid., 61.
8. Ibid., 233.
9. Ibid., 233–34.
10. Ibid., 236–37.
11. Ibid., 2.
12. Rieff, *Freud: The Mind of the Moralist*, 377.
13. Rieff, *Triumph of the Therapeutic.*
14. Bellah et al., *Habits of the Heart,* 64.
15. Lichterman, *The Search for Political Community.*
16. For the Greens, an activist group in Lichterman's study that was noted for its personalized or self-expressive politics, the goal was to sustain a commitment and togetherness *among* people with individualized, diverse radicalization experiences (p. 66).
17. Alexis de Tocqueville, *Democracy in America*, edited and abridged by Richard D. Heffner (New York: Signet Classic, 2001), 153–54.
18. Rieff, *Triumph of the Therapeutic.*

Chapter Eight

Lifting Up the Carpet, Opening Doors, and Reintegration

HONEST BODIES, REAL BODIES, AND RECLAIMING THE SPIRIT OF AFRICAN-AMERICAN GLBT WORSHIPPERS

The purpose of the therapeutic ethic is to generate a sense of well-being through the living of life itself,[1] but well-being and "good living" require first that people resolve major life conflicts. For congregation members at Unity Fellowship Church, this requires, first, finding a church that will allow them to worship openly as GLBT, African-American Christians. Required religious elements necessarily affirm the sexual orientation of GLBT people, doing so explicitly in sermons, but they also must affirm the congregation members' other social statuses too, including their status as black men and women with deep religious roots. By affirming congregation members wholly, Unity Fellowship Church and its therapeutic form of religion empower congregation members to "reclaim the spirit,"[2] by enabling the expressions of what Patricia Hills Collins calls "honest bodies."[3]

In *Black Sexual Politics,* Collins stipulated at least five requirements of "honest bodies." First, honest bodies "strive to treat the mental, spiritual, and physical aspects of living as human beings as interactive and synergistic," rather than prioritizing one element over the other. Second, developing honest bodies and a politics grounded in that fact begins from the inside out. That is, the emphasis is (or should be) placed on how "honest Black bodies feel, hear, and move," rather than on how black bodies appear and how others interpret them. In other words, the focus should be on how individuals themselves *actually* experience their bodies, not how others see their bodies. Third, an honest body is one that is "in touch with its life spirit, or soul."[4] Fourth, honest bodies are sexually autonomous, and the sexual autonomy extends to both straight black and gay black people alike; both are permitted to engage in various forms of sexual expression that bring them pleasure and joy. For black gay men and women, in particular, the honest body means not having to separate the body from the self, as well as the freedom to pursue one's own sense of the erotic.[5]

Finally, Collins maintains that attaining honest bodies necessarily requires an expanded body politics, which means a new understanding of sexuality that integrates the ideas of soul and embodiment. This is necessitated, according to Collins, because sexuality "lies at the intersection of soul (individual expressiveness) and body (dance and movement)." To enable this, however, requires a rethinking of sexual autonomy for black people that "rejoins mind, soul, and body."[6]

McGuire's definition of "real bodies" aligns with Collins' definition of "honest bodies," but encompasses more corporeal elements. In particular, "real bodies," according to McGuire, includes bodies of all types—both healthy and unhealthy bodies, athletic and frail bodies, pregnant bodies, arthritic bodies, malnourished bodies, obese bodies, and suffering bodies. "Real bodies" also include bodies that create and destroy, as well as "bodies that nurse and bodies that torture the bodies of others."[7] Human embodiment, distinct from "real bodies," is the physical behaviors intimately identified with real human, material bodies. The behaviors include basic human functions such as eating and sleeping, but also include the more "invisible" human functions, such as defecating, sweating, and having sex.[8]

Religion enters the picture of the real body in that humans are not disembodied spirits.[9] That is, according to Wade Clark Roof, we are unable to know ourselves apart from our bodies.[10] Hence, it should come as no surprise that our physical body plays a prominent role in our spiritual quests. Indeed, spiritual seekers may talk about "reclaiming" their (devalued) bodies during their spiritual journeys. Presumably, their bodily recovery occurs simultaneously with their spiritual discovery. At this point, spiritual seekers, having gained acceptance of their bodies, come to feel better about their bodies. They then begin to feel better about themselves in the general sense. In this sense spirituality and embodiment are intimately linked, with the well-being of one associated with the well-being of the other.[11]

Enabling sexual autonomy for GLBT, African-American Christians, thus, is not simply a cognitive process; it involves far more than paying lip service to worshippers who happen to be GLBT. To truly enable sexual autonomy, religious authority must speak a language that incorporates both physical bodies ("real bodies") and human embodiment—in this case, recognizing that the act of sex is a part of "real" human bodies and real human lives. By explicitly acknowledging, as well as affirming, their sexual bodies, by allowing open sexual expressions, and by linking their sexuality to their lives as black GLBT men and women, Archbishop Bean and his church are helping to integrate congregation members' mind, spirit, and bodies to form a complete whole. In doing so, Archbishop Bean has unlocked the shackles that have long restricted black bodies and, more specifically, black GLBT bodies. The social control of black GLBT bodies has at last returned to their rightful owners, rather than subject to the whims of religion and other social institutions.

The religious integration of GLBT black men and women is particularly arduous because it involves a struggle for the full humanity of GLBT black men and women, which necessarily involves the embodiment and expressions of black bodies—*sexual* black bodies. Open expressions of GLBT sexuality signifies that the church has overcome "fixed and overdetermined identities."[12] As this case study has highlighted, the integration process of religious black GLBT men and women is not easy. It requires a religion that, in fact, links theology to real material human bodies and not simply to abstract ideas or ideals. A religion that truly allows its adherents to be autonomous must incorporate "real bodies" and all the functions and behaviors associated with real human bodies. If we are not disembodied spirits, then our bodies cannot be severed from our minds and souls, or from our spirituality (or religion). In the same vein, the behaviors associated with real bodies—which includes the physical act of intercourse—cannot be severed from our minds and souls, because they are what we do, and help shape the basis of who we are.

GENDER, HUMAN SEXUALITY, AND RELIGION: THE LINK BETWEEN SEXISM AND HOMOPHOBIA

Religious institutions' stance on gender matters, because gender and sexuality inextricably are linked. Homophobia works effectively as a weapon of sexism because it functions in congruence with heterosexism, an institutionalized set of behaviors and beliefs that presume that heterosexuality is the only acceptable form of sexual expression.[13] Heterosexism creates the climate for homophobia by assuming that the world is and must be heterosexual;[14] that is, the norm is heterosexual, and those who are not heterosexual are "abnormal" or "deviant." This is known as compulsory heterosexuality, what Adrienne Rich refers to as ideology and institutionalized practices that demand heterosexuality.[15]

According to feminist scholar Adrienne Rich, heterosexuality is "both forcibly and subliminally imposed"[16] by a society's social institutions. Specifically, compulsory heterosexuality is backed by institutions such as religion and marriage, both of which encourage rigid gender divisions, procreation, and the notion of the nuclear family as normative, if not ideal. To go against these social expectations would be considered deviant and problemat-

ic. Thus, adults (adult women in particular) who remain single and uncou-
pled are ridiculed, and women who love other women and men who love
other men are seen as sexually pathological.[17]

According to Suzanne Pharr, gay men and lesbians are considered threats
to male dominance and control, albeit in slightly different ways. Lesbians are
perceived as women who can live without men and, therefore, are believed to
be anti-men. The lesbian is seen as a threat to the nuclear family, the bastion
of patriarchy. In contrast, gay men are not viewed as anti-men but rather they
are perceived as insufficiently masculine. Gay men's expressions of physical
affection, bonding, and romantic love with other men outside the context of
sports and war suggest that they are not "real men." Because they are not
considered real men, gay men therefore are perceived as being more similar
to women and are identified with women. Like women, gay men therefore
must be dominated.[18] And like lesbians, gay men threaten norms related to
sex role differentiation, as well as threaten the nuclear family ideal. Because
they are threats to the status quo, gay men (and lesbians) must be contained,
sanctioned, and suppressed.

These outcomes underscore how heterosexism and homophobia both
function as systems of social control. That is, failure to conform to normative
heterosexist expectations may lead to sanctions that range from ridicule to
ostracism to violence.[19] The process further draws attention to the linkage
between sex and sexual orientation and, more specifically, sexism and homophobia: Homophobia ultimately represents a rejection of femininity/effemi-
nacy. In rejecting all things feminine, homophobia provides support for masculine power and men's dominance of women.

Contesting and eradicating homophobia, thus, necessarily involves a contestation and eradication of sexist systems. This is where religious organizations play a role. As major agents of socialization, religious organizations are
central in teaching and disseminating values, ideas, and practices related to
intergroup relations. Congregations are therefore integral in helping shape
people's position on gender relations.

While black churches remain key symbols of strength and social change
for African Americans, their stance on gender equality is inconsistent. Sandra
Barnes notes that while black churches remain activist, social activism does
not necessarily correlate positively with support for sex/gender equality, as
other social justice issues (e.g., racism) tend to take precedence. Factors that
do seem to positively correlate with sex/gender equality, as measured
through support for women in the pastorate, include: black liberation theology, womanist theology, and clergy involvement in social justice issues. In
Barnes' study, there were also indications of denominational differences,
with Baptists least likely to support sex/gender equality.[20] The literatures
also suggest that increased representation of women in the congregations, as

well as an increased presence of progressive male clergy, may help facilitate greater gender egalitarianism.[21]

Audre Lorde maintained that we have been programmed to handle difference in one of three ways: 1) ignore it; 2) copy it, if we think it is dominant; or 3) destroy it if we think it is subordinate.[22] The founder and clergy of Unity Fellowship Church, however, do not handle difference in any of these three ways. Rather, they welcome and celebrate differences, and they encourage the fluidity and multiplicity of gender, sexuality, and other meaning systems, a stark contrast to more traditional churches, which tend to be constrained by a normative framework that emphasizes heterosexuality, monogamy, marriage, and family, and which tend to advocate an ethic of sexual control. The clergy at Unity Fellowship Church stress the normalcy of gender and sexual variations.

Simultaneously, the clergy at Unity Fellowship Church appear to rely on three major strategies to destabilize and subvert gender and sexual categories: 1) redefinition; 2) legitimation; and 3) resistance. Consistent with Oswald's definition, "redefinition" includes "paradigmatic or meaning-making strategies that create linguistic and symbolic structures to affirm one's network."[23] At Unity Fellowship Church, oppressive biblical passages and religious themes are reinterpreted in ways that are non-oppressive to the GLBT community, women, and people of color. God, for instance, is defined as neither male nor female. Instead, the god at Unity Fellowship Church "is spirit and spirit has no gender." In worship services, Archbishop Bean, a male, often refers to God as either a "She" or a spirit that is neither male nor female. At one particular worship service, Archbishop Bean asserted, "God is love. I didn't say a man. I didn't say a woman. God is love." In both worship services and Bible study classes, Archbishop Bean even has prolonged the enunciation of "she" when referring to God; his intention was to "jar some of us," "wake us up," and to get the congregation to realize that masculinity need not dominate, even in the religious setting.[24]

Legitimation incorporates strategies that support non-normative relationships. This includes the conscious creation, ritualization, and legalization of these same non-normative relationships.[25] Increasing the presence and visibility of women leadership is one key legitimation strategy. This is especially important in religious organizations, in which institutional power tends to be organized by both gender and sexuality. Heterosexual males most often occupy the most visible roles and leadership positions in the religious setting, with women often relegated to the supportive church roles.[26] In this way, the church organization resembles the larger organization of both labor and society, with males monopolizing the more visible, higher-authority, and more valuable positions.

Although he is male, Archbishop Bean is fully cognizant of the gender disparity in religious leadership roles. Because of this awareness, he makes it a special point to increase the presence and visibility of the female clergy at his church, a sharp contrast to more traditional African-American churches, in which the male clergy seem to dominate the visible leadership positions and women clergy are rarely, if at all, seen *at* the pulpit and/or presiding over sermons.[27] An entire month is even dedicated to celebrate womanhood; at Unity, March is deemed "Women's Herstory Month." During this month, the women clergy and male-to-female transgender individuals are celebrated, and they provide the spiritual messages in worship services.

Another way in which Archbishop Bean legitimizes womanhood and, black womanhood/sisterhood in particular, is through frequent reminders of the pivotal roles women played in both within-group (African-American) and general human survival. He underscored the different forms of labor women undertake: physical labor, emotional labor, and reproductive labor. In all, Archbishop Bean regularly underscores women's self-sacrifices for the betterment of man, community, and society.

At Unity Fellowship Church, legitimation is perhaps most exemplified in the institutionalization of same-sex marriage ceremonies within the religious organization, even during a period when same-sex marriage was not yet recognized by the legislature, the courts, and the public. Legitimation at Unity Fellowship Church also involved the creation of external support systems (e.g., support groups and meetings) to help individuals manage non-normative forms of gender and sexual identities both within and outside of the church.

Finally, at all times there is resistance, deliberate and intentional actions that openly challenge and oppose the status quo. This is illustrated by: Archbishop Bean's and other clergy's calling attention to various systems of oppression; their recognition of GLBT women and men as not aberrant but as a legitimate, "socially normal" group of people; organized political marches and demonstrations; and, of course, the initial creation of their separatist church. Perhaps most importantly, rather than construing the body—notably women's body and the homosexual body—as impediments to sanctification, the church founder and clergy of Unity Fellowship Church view women and GLBT persons as holy, sacred bodies, rather than sinful, profane ones.

LIBERATION THEOLOGY AND A LIBERATION OF A PEOPLE

Religious ideology and teachings are important in manufacturing and reconstructing ideologies and, in many instances, reinforcing hegemonic power. The significance of hegemonic power, according to Patricia Hill Collins, lies in its ability to shape consciousness through the manipulation of ideas, images, symbols, and ideologies.[28] In this way, theology helps define gender roles in the church, and what constitutes appropriate sexuality. Thus, theology potentially can be oppressive or liberating.

Unity Fellowship Church's theological approach is one of openness, tolerance, inclusiveness, and affirmation of differences. The church founder and clergy welcome and celebrate differences, and accept the fluidity and multiplicity of gender, sexuality, and other meanings, including in the belief and understanding of God, religion, and spirituality. In Unity Fellowship Church's orientation brochure, God is defined as neither male nor female: "God is spirit and spirit has no gender." And God, regardless of form, is everywhere present, in multiple forms. And regardless of form and specific faith, God is equated with love; that is to say, love is the metaphor for God. Love is grounded in the acceptance and embracing of all, regardless of person, and love is exemplified in practices that include advancing the well-being of the community and general society, advocating for social justice, and providing for those in need.

Archbishop Bean and his clergy describe their church theology as "liberation theology," because it is a theology that frees the oppressed. It is a theology that is: not male-dominated; not oppressive to women; not just European in scope; not oppressive to lesbian and gay people; and not oppressive to poor people or to those with a positive HIV serostatus. In other words, Unity Fellowship Church's theology frees people from the shame and anguish associated with their marginalized statuses. Instead, there are celebrations of these social statuses, particularly with respect to sexual orientation. The following is typical of a message put forth from the pulpit:

> There has been no mistake. No mistakes have been made. You are just who you are supposed to be today. Now celebrate your sexual orientation whether you are having sex or not. Realize the choice is yours, so celebrate right now. Your sexual orientation is a blessing!

Because the religious leaders at Unity Fellowship Church are multiply marginalized, just as their parishioners are, they are able to transform their church from what might have been a closed structure to an open one. They do so by re-defining the goals of religion and spirituality, and re-interpreting religion in ways that address their parishioners' unique needs, doing so in a manner that empowers all individuals, rather than simply a select, privileged few. In large part, this involves parsing biblical passages, understanding the context in which the Bible was written, and understanding that the Bible is man-made. As such, it is not inerrant; indeed, the religious text is open to questioning, critique, and re-interpretation, as well as open to modernization.

WHY UNITY FELLOWSHIP CHURCH MATTERS

The founder of Unity Fellowship Church recognized the theological crisis of wanting to maintain the viability or plausibility of a church in an environment that may not accept its traditional religious definitions of "reality," particularly in the age of AIDS. One response to this theological crisis is through accommodation, which Berger maintains involves the reorganization of the religious institution in order to make it more relevant to the modern world.[29] Accommodating tactics, however, suggests an obligingness to certain population segments, or attempts to reconcile differences between two or more groups. Archbishop Bean found accommodating strategies insufficient and, accordingly, engaged in more deliberate and intentional actions, openly opposing the status quo.

Unity Fellowship Church represents an oppositional religious culture. Created in response to the AIDS epidemic specifically, Archbishop Bean established a separate, autonomous religious organization for African Americans in urban areas who were gay/lesbian/bisexual/transgender and/or HIV-positive. The creation of this alternative worship site enabled a safe space to worship, new opportunity structures, the development of indigenous leadership, and critical reflection, allowing organizational members to interpret and articulate their own unique experiences and meanings free from the imposition of ideological and moral presuppositions of dominant groups.[30]

The religious leaders of these alternative or emerging religions tend to be open and honest—even transparent about their faith, struggles, and commitments—and the members of these religious communities tend to be true to their convictions not because of what their parents believed, or what society and mainstream religious institutions have dictated to them, but because they have actively appropriated the convictions as their own.[31] Autonomous churches such as Unity Fellowship Church, thus, come to represent the "authentic church" of HIV-positive, GLBT, African-American individuals.

Within the Unity Fellowship Church structure, Archbishop Bean has created systems of self-valuation and self-definition that address the special needs of congregation members. In particular, Archbishop Bean has replaced externally derived images and belief systems with systems that are authentic to the GLBT, poverty-stricken, HIV+, spiritual African Americans.

But beyond the cultural affirmations, Unity Fellowship Church matters to its members because this church allows members to define religion in ways that are meaningful to them, and it allows them to define for themselves who they are and what they want out of life, without having other people's demands imposed upon them. A personalized form of religion that is highly therapeutically oriented enables this. A personalized form of religion, at least in the case of Unity Fellowship Church, allows a high degree of flexibility in interpreting scriptures, sermons, and religious symbols. Archbishop Bean does not impose any specific beliefs on church members. He does not impose on them a single definition of religion, spirituality, God, and other religious concepts/symbols, and there is no requirement that congregation members are to embrace Archbishop Bean's versions. Indeed, Archbishop Bean encourages congregation members to approach God and religion through their own lens.

This flexibility in the interpretation of religion is crucial, because it allows congregation members to self-define religion on their own terms. But it also allows congregation members to define who they are as individuals, and as a group of people. Kyla underscored the importance of this ability to self-define. She noted that other churches to which congregation members belonged to, or visited, tended to label them as problematic and as needing help. As she stated, "[T]hey assume that who you are is a problem. Because that's how they choose to define us. And Unity has [taught] me that you don't get to define who I am. You don't have the authority to define who I am. I define myself for me." For congregation members at Unity, then, their religion—a therapeutic form of religion—includes the power to recognize themselves as "not ungodly . . . not unmerciful . . . and not idol worshippers," but rather "a holy homosexual."

That Archbishop Bean allows congregation members to self-define religion appears inconsistent with the conceptualization of religion as a shared system of beliefs and practices. Yet, the inconsistencies vanish if we recognize that at Unity Fellowship Church, personalized or individualized forms of religion represent the shared way of thinking and doing things. Thus, in spite of seemingly disparate interpretive religious schemes, we see that these interpretive schemes are not so disparate after all, as they all seek to uplift and affirm the social and religious identities and lives of GLBT worshippers through therapeutic means. Congregation members at Unity Fellowship Church strive to transform religion in order to (re)gain some control over their own lives. They therefore incorporate their own self-definition of what religion is and encompasses, in ways that incorporate their sexual identities.

TRANSFORMATION, SELF-DISCOVERY, AND SPIRITUAL ENLIGHTENMENT

Therapeutic religion matters because it provides a springboard toward self-betterment and transformation. The respondents in this study see therapeutic religion as valuable to the extent that it helps them make sense of their own experiences. It helps them make sense of religion, and it helps them understand the world around them. More broadly, therapeutic religion matters to the respondents in this study because it enhances their well-being. While (psychological) well-being cannot be empirically measured in this study, the respondents' assessments of their own transformations are loose ways of measuring the efficacy of therapeutic religion, at least at Unity Fellowship Church.

For some of the respondents I interviewed, the openness, the supportive environment, and the accepting outlook of Unity Fellowship Church have enabled them to openly proclaim their attraction for same-sex partners and, in some cases, to openly announce their HIV status. For others, Unity Fellowship Church has provided a safe place to worship. These allowances are substantial for many of the congregation members at Unity, who were raised in churches that had very rigid gender divisions and that were homophobic.

Some of the respondents noted how the cultural strategies have been life-altering. For Raymond, who is HIV-positive and a recovering alcoholic and drug addict, Unity has taught him how to "love myself. Accept who I am. Not worry about what other people think about me." In her trajectory at Unity, Shelly mustered the courage to openly disclose her HIV status, although it required an eight-year "healing process" as a church member and the need to first "grow through a lot of stuff" before she was able to do so.

On the surface, it may appear that therapeutic religion is simply about the individual. Critics such as Philip Rieff, in fact, argued that therapeutic societies are self-centered and even narcissistic.[32] But spirituality has always centered on the individual. In *After Heaven: Spirituality in America Since the 1950s*, Robert Wuthnow[33] points out the close and complex relationship between spirituality and the inner self. One of his respondents, a survivor of spousal abuse, discovered that her recovery from abuse required that she not only re-evaluate her outlook on life, but that she also engage in introspective activities. These activities were necessary in order to understand what was going on inside her, and to allow her to more fully understand, and appreciate, her emotions. As she was recovering emotionally, Wuthnow's respondent found that simultaneously her spirituality deepened; she found that her relationship with God was a source of inner strength and was what kept her sane.[34]

Other respondents in Wuthnow's work similarly underwent dual journeys of self-discovery and spiritual-discovery as they confronted personal crises. Spirituality, however, focused mainly on who an individual was, and what the individual wanted out of life. Hence, the spiritual journey was very much linked to introspection and "finding oneself." A successful search culminated in self-discovery and, perhaps not coincidently, a heightened and more intense relationship with one's God.

Similarly, for congregation members at Unity Fellowship Church, the journey wasn't entirely about their psychological states. Some of the respondents in my study focused on their relationship with their God, and they expressed a need to find a comfortable "fit" in the relationship. "Fit" implied that they were so comfortable in their spiritual skin that they were willing to surrender to their God, entrusting God wholly, and simply letting their God take control of their life.

The difference between the self-discovery journey and the spiritual journey, hence, is that the latter journey transcends emotions and feelings. The spiritual journey requires that a person come to terms with: what s/he believes God represents, what s/he believes religion represents, and his/her relationship with each. Nonetheless, the spiritual journey commonly coincides with the journey toward self-discovery, in which a person takes a mental inventory of his or her life, and then assesses it in light of what s/he wants out of life. In this respect, it is virtually impossible to disentangle the self-discovery journey from the spiritual journey. Complicating matters is the blurring of the boundaries between therapy and religion. As Robert Wuthnow aptly stated in *After Heaven*, "The blending of language from psychology, therapy, and recovery literature with the language of religion makes it difficult to determine whether spirituality of the inner self is similar to traditional religion or a radical departure from it."[35]

With histories of trauma and lifestyles considered non-normative, traditional religious teachings and doctrines simply were not feasible sources for spiritual inspiration and enlightenment for congregation members at Unity Fellowship Church. Religion and spirituality had to make sense on their own terms, and they had to be rooted in their lived experiences. Given this context, it is not surprising that congregation members at Unity underwent a simultaneous dual journey toward self-discovery and spiritual discovery. The two journeys necessarily were concurrent, because the spiritual journey had to reflect a person's changing understandings of the self, particularly with respect to how the self relates to larger society.

The interview respondents in this study, in fact, revealed that self-discovery and spirituality discovery most often coincided. In the periods they were "shopping" for churches, some of the respondents expressed doubts about religion and about organized religion in particular. Some respondents even expressed uneasiness about what they observed were contradictions in their God. Most often, they wondered how a loving God could inflict pain, suffering, and even consign people to hell.

During this period of spiritual questioning, it seemed as though the respondents were also simultaneously unsure about their own position in society, about where they fit in society, if they even fit, as homosexual Christians. During this period, they began to embark on a journey of self-discovery. It was only when they reached a self-understanding, and a self-acceptance of their GLBT or HIV-status, did they also reach a comfortable relationship with their God. Hence, for congregation members at Unity, a "deeper" spirituality is harvested only through a better understanding of themselves. That is to say, the journey involves a "quest to overcome estrangement," which Wuthnow notes is "an important part of many Americans' search for a spirituality that gives them a new sense of self."[36]

Minister Pepper illustrates this dual process. She described being "born again" when she found Unity Fellowship Church. She explained that she underwent a period in which she would have "quiet time," whether in a public space or in her own home, where she would meditate. The meditation, which she learned at one of the church's Wednesday-night spiritual renewal classes, helped her to understand what it meant "to pray and talk to God." She recalled always questioning the meaning of things, and always hungry for knowledge during this period of spiritual discovery. She described it as an awkward phase, in which she felt like a baby, and sensed that everything around her was new and unfamiliar. But gradually she came to learn how to meditate, and to learn "how to *really* pray." "Real praying," for Minister Pepper, meant that she could "talk" to God, converse with Him, and understand that God is always right beside her.

But "being born again," at least for Minister Pepper, meant not only spiritual re-discovery, but a personal renewal. She explained that her spiritual discovery has led her to make changes in her personal life. In particular, she now lives "for this moment" and tries not to worry about yesterday. This ability to "stay in the moment" is one that she previously lacked, as her mind would wander and she would ruminate on the past. Her newfound relationship with God, and understanding the meaning of prayer, however, have taught Minister Pepper to simply live in the present and "[t]hank God for the moment, because the moment is really all we have. We're not promised the next second."

Candy provided a more concrete example of how the spiritual journey often coincides with the journey toward self-discovery. She spoke of "cleansing the spirit," which was associated with a re-examination of one's life. Indeed, she equated the enlightenment she received through introspection and a subsequent discovery that she is "worthy" of having fulfilling and healthy relationships that are free of verbal and physical abuse to spiritual enlightenment. This self-discovery allowed her to extricate herself from unhealthy relationships and provided her "the power to make changes." This epiphany, which she found on Sunday from Archbishop Bean, was also what impelled her to seek a sex change. As she explained:

> I felt like [Archbishop Bean] was preaching about being your true self. And I felt like I wasn't my true self, and I felt like I was deceiving myself and I was deceiving everybody else, and I felt like, how can I go on with this masquerade? I need to be who I really am. . . . I remember him preaching about being your true self, being true to yourself, and that kind of thing. And that kind of struck me.

Thereafter, Candy explored her options for the surgical procedure. On referral from a friend, she traveled to Thailand for the sex-change procedure. Accompanying her on the trip was a filmmaker, who recorded Candy's transition in a documentary film.

Archbishop Bean's sermon messages provided the stimulus for Candy's spiritual and personal journeys, because his messages resonated like no other religious messages had. There was an emotional element to Archbishop Bean's messages, and they were so personal and timely—so much so that Candy described coming home from worship services and just crying in her bedroom. Archbishop Bean's sermons were emotionally cathartic for Candy. She explained:

> I was like, "Wow!" I can't believe that, you know, the things that I heard and everything. And it really touched me and it made me feel at home. And I felt like he [Archbishop Bean] really knew who I was. And I felt like I was hiding. And I felt like I had been hiding for years and years. Once I figured out who I truly was . . . 'cause for a long time, I didn't know who I was. And so, it was okay where I was. But when I realized who I was, and it wasn't who I was portraying myself to be, then that was where the dilemma came. I said, "Okay, I need to be who I am. I need to make me happy." And so, I did. And I'm glad. I'm very happy that . . . I feel like my life has been a journey, and that I've been put on this path to do things, and you gotta do 'em in that order. And I did that and I did that, and I did that. And the time came for me to have the surgery, and I did that. And this is like a journey. So it's not. . . . It was not like I'm going to ever get to a goal. I think this is just a journey to walk through.

Both the journey toward self-discovery and the spiritual journey proved to be challenging for the congregation members at Unity Fellowship Church. The path toward self-discovery and spiritual discovery often was not linear, nor instantaneous. Ramona narrated how problematic her own journey was. Her biggest challenge toward self-discovery was learning how to love herself. Although she indicated that she has moved forward, particularly when compared to her location seven years ago, "It's still a work in progress." Spiritually, she indicated that she was "constantly" thrown in situations in which was personally challenged, and her faith was challenged as well. She indicated that she resolved these challenges by simply putting herself out there and giving in to God. She asserted confidently, "I actually believe that He'll take care of it in his time."

When I pointed out to Ramona that it sounded as though she has achieved a degree of peace of mind, she concurred. She went on to explain that her journey toward self-discovery and her spiritual journey allowed her to have peace of mind "in my home, my life, my work. Whenever I'm in a relationship, I have it there too. When I don't have those things, I take care of them because I love me. I love God first, then I love me. So, I don't let anything get in the way of those two things." In this statement, she alludes to the inseparability of the spirituality and her inner self. But when she emphasizes, "I love God first, then I love me," she is asserting how spirituality—that is, her relationship with God—precedes all else in importance.

Some critics might find the type of spiritual journeys that the interview respondents described to be far too inward- or self-oriented. These critics might describe congregation members at Unity Fellowship Church as searching for God too much inside themselves, rather than relying more heavily on more authoritative sources for spiritual direction—religious traditions and theology, for instance. However, the respondents in this study indicated that they still need religious traditions and theology, despite engaging in what appears to be very inward-oriented quests. Indeed, this is why they come to Unity Fellowship Church: They needed to be involved in a religious community in which participants, too, were searching for themselves, and searching for spiritual enlightenment. It wasn't simply about looking inside themselves and relying on themselves as the sole source of religious authority, in spite of relying heavily on themselves and their own experiences as the source of "truth." They were also searching for a community and, more specifically, a religious home that permitted multiple "truths."

In this regard, the experiences of the respondents seem to resemble the process that Wuthnow noted in *After Heaven*. Wuthnow suggested that the therapeutic language that characterizes 12-step and other supportive communities are concerned with finding truth through increased awareness of the self. Self-awareness, however, is facilitated through the participation in a supportive community. That is to say, self-awareness is unlikely to be effective without membership in a like-minded community that will support the person's efforts.[37]

A STEPPING STONE TOWARD A BETTER TOMORROW

To be sure, Unity Fellowship Church is first a religious organization. But secondarily, it is a domain for adult resocialization. Much like a 12-step support group, Unity Fellowship Church attempts to reintegrate individuals into mainstream society by reorienting them psychologically and spiritually. The purpose of this congregation's form of religion is to help people feel better, and help them function in healthier, more effective, and more productive ways. But for "non-normals," therapeutic religion also aims to help them feel normal.

The healing process at Unity Fellowship Church combines various therapeutic rituals that range from repetition of affirmations to affective and embodied rituals. But healing itself cannot be time-tabled; it is an extremely individualized process that, for congregation members, requires both self-discovery and spiritual growth. What do these processes entail? They require emotional healing, which, above all, means that congregation members need to learn to love themselves. Indeed, "learning to love oneself" is a message that is reiterated at Unity Fellowship Church with great frequency, and it is the hope of the church pastor that when congregation members learn to love themselves, they aspire and work for a better life, and work to improve themselves and others. The belief is that with self-love and acceptance, congregation members will become more autonomous and more integrated into society. And as they become more self-empowered in the process, the hope is that they will learn to resist labels and messages imposed upon them by others.

But the recovery process necessarily is a spiritual one, for successful recovery occurs when a person has reclaimed God. Recovery means that the individual is finally able to conceive of God as a force inside himself, rather than as an external force over which he has no control. Recovery involves gaining the ability to see God as part of the self, which means that the individual must have control of his own life. That is to say, recovery means reclaiming one's inner strength or soul, which represents God and God's spirit and strength.

For congregation members, Unity Fellowship Church is a part of a long journey toward self-discovery, spiritual enlightenment, and healing. Because the journey is long, with unpredictable twists and turns, for some people, Unity is an intermediary or a stepping stone toward something bigger. As congregation members heal, some may leave this church and return to their former congregations; others may transfer to different congregations—often larger, more well-funded congregations, whether GLBT-centered or not.[38]

But it appears that a defining moment in the lives of these former members is that Unity Fellowship Church contributed to their recovery, through messages of affirmation and self-acceptance, and through unwavering displays of love and acceptance. The strategy is distinctly therapeutic, but deceptively simple. Reverend Redd summed it up best when I asked him how Unity Fellowship Church reconciled the dilemma that demands that they provide services and care for the same people that religious traditions teach them to reject. He responded:

> I think the way they reconcile it is through the simple concept of L-O-V-E. . . . I mean there's a text that says that, "First love the Lord, thy God, with all thy heart, thy mind, thy soul." And the second is liken to "Love thy neighbor as thyself." . . . To me it becomes no more a dilemma [chuckles], because. . . . Not that it doesn't become a dilemma, but you don't have to reconcile it when you recognize that the only way to respond to someone in pain is through love. What is there to reconcile?

It dawned on me from Reverend Redd's response that I, as the researcher, had assumed that there was a dilemma or contradiction in the first place. I also assumed that the clergy necessarily respond to religious contradictions through revisions of sacred texts and traditions. Never in my mind did it cross my mind that the solution for harmonizing congregation members' religious and sexual and other social identities was so obvious: through the demonstration of love. This means accepting and affirming people as they are, with their flaws and dark pasts and all, and letting them grow and heal on their own time.

The interview respondents, in fact, consistently described Unity as "accepting" and "non-judgmental." The element of acceptance, according to Rose, is a crucial part of recovery:

> To me, they [Unity Fellowship Church clergy and members] respect me, even though they know my history. And they accept me. They don't put any . . . chains or anything across the doorway when I get ready to come in. They're not locking down stuff in the church when I walk in. And that makes me feel good. So they are accepting me, and acceptance is a big part for a recovering addict.

In this respect, Unity Fellowship Church contains a prominent characteristic of the "seeker churches" that Kimon Howland Sargeant identified: There is an absence of judgmental or discriminatory behavior that singles out behaviors or people deemed to be unacceptable or immoral.[39] Suspending moral judgments cannot be underestimated enough, especially for the traumatized lot that characterizes the members of Unity Fellowship Church.

Kyla suggested that many people arrive at the doorsteps of Unity Fellowship Church with various issues, including "serious mental health issues . . . dual, triple, and quadruple diagnosed with HIV—a lot of problems," and Unity is "the first place that has embraced them, let them . . . help them to understand some of those issues that they're going through, or motivating them to go get help for some of those issues." She added that despite all of these "issues" that people bring with them to Unity:

> [W]e [at Unity Fellowship Church] have fun with people and we don't treat people any—they [the clergy] don't seem to treat people any differently, you know. Those people seem to come and they can [be themselves]. . . . It's an environment they can feel comfortable in that they can be . . . accepted. And participate in and be engaged.

The timespan for growth and healing is indefinite. It may take years for congregation members to acquire the self-awareness they need for both personal and spiritual growth. Or it may take a lifetime. The power of Unity Fellowship Church, thus, is that, in spite of the vacillations among individual members' lives, this church is a source of stability, steadiness, and, always, a source for reassurance, compassion, and love. These elements were absent at other congregations to which Unity Fellowship Church members belonged, or at least visited, even if only briefly. Congregation members may enter and exit Unity Fellowship Church during their quests for self-discovery and spiritual discovery, but what is certain is that Unity Fellowship Church has, in some way, shaped their journeys positively, and has come to symbolize a spiritual home to which people are always welcome to return to at any time.

NOTES

1. Betsworth, *Social Ethics*, 106.
2. David Shallenberger, *Reclaiming the Spirit: Gay Men and Women Come to Terms with Religion* (New Brunswick, NJ: Rutgers University Press, 1998).
3. Patricia Hill Collins, *Black Sexual Politics: African Americans, Gender, and the New Racism* (New York: Routledge, 2004).
4. Ibid., 283.
5. Ibid., 287.
6. Ibid., 286.
7. Meredith B. McGuire, "Why Bodies Matter: A Sociological Reflection on Spirituality and Materiality," *Spiritus* 3, no.1 (2003): 1.
8. Ibid.
9. Ibid., 15.
10. Roof, *Spiritual Marketplace*, 105.
11. Ibid.
12. Anthony B. Pinn, "Black Bodies in Pain and Ecstasy: Terror, Subjectivity, and the Nature of Black Religion," *Nova Religio: The Journal of Alternative and Emergent Religions* 7, no. 1 (2003): 83.
13. Margaret L. Andersen, *Thinking about Women: Sociological Perspectives on Sex and Gender*, 5th ed. (Boston: Allyn and Bacon, 2000), 94.
14. Suzanne Pharr, *Homophobia: A Weapon of Sexism* (Berkeley, CA: Chardon Press, 1997), 16.
15. Adrienne Rich, "Compulsory Heterosexuality and Lesbian Existence," *Signs* 5, no. 4 (1980).
16. Ibid., 653.
17. Andersen, *Thinking about Women*, 84.
18. Pharr, *Homophobia*, 18–19.
19. Ibid., 94.
20. Sandra L. Barnes, "Whosoever Will Let Her Come: Social Activism and Gender Inclusivity in the Black Church," *Journal for the Scientific Study of Religion* 45, no. 3 (2006): 379.
21. Ibid., 372.
22. Audre Lorde, "Age, Race, Class and Sex: Women Redefining Difference," in *Gender Through the Prism of Difference*, 2nd ed., eds. Maxine Baca Zinn, Pierrette Hondagneu-Sotelo, and Michael A. Messner (reprint, Needham Heights, MA: Allyn & Bacon, [1984] 2000), 503.
23. Ramona Faith Oswald, "Resilience within the Family Networks of Lesbians and Gay Men: Intentionality and Redefinition," *Journal of Marriage and Family* 64, no. 2 (2002): 381.
24. Regardless of whether the context is religious or secular, even socially progressive individuals, feminists, and women themselves continue to refer to God as a "He." Archbishop Bean attributed this phenomenon to long-ingrained ideas that belittle and subordinate women, which make it very difficult for people to link women with the divine.
25. Ibid.

26. Cheryl Townsend Gilkes, "The Roles of Church and Community Mothers: Ambivalent American Sexism or Fragmented African Familyhood," *Journal of Feminist Studies in Religion* 2, no. 1 (1986): 41–59.

27. Because Archbishop Carl Bean is the founder of the Unity Fellowship Church movement, no other clergy in this movement, whether male or female, will surpass him in terms of visibility or power.

28. Collins, *Black Feminist Thought*, 284–85.

29. Berger, *The Sacred Canopy.*

30. Dwight B. Billings, "Religion as Opposition: A Gramscian Analysis," *American Journal of Sociology* 96, no. 1 (1990): 27.

31. Sargeant, *Seeker Churches*, 166.

32. Rieff, *Triumph of the Therapeutic.*

33. Wuthnow, *After Heaven.*

34. Ibid., 144.

35. Ibid., 157.

36. Ibid., 166.

37. Ibid., 154.

38. Reverend Linda notes that people tend to have a habit of separating themselves once they have "made it." Part of this is because they may not want to be reminded, or be associated with, people who have not made it, because it reminds them of who they once were, in a period in which they were struggling. But she also pointed out that despite some members' departure from Unity, some people still periodically return to Unity, particularly if they are experiencing personal crises or are in trouble. In this regard, Unity still is "home" to the people who have "healed" and have outgrown Unity.

39. Sargeant, *Seeker Churches*, 104–5.

Chapter Nine

Pain, the Truth of Human Feelings, and the Need for Therapeutic Religion

To combat both the fear- and hate-mongering rhetoric that characterizes many traditional religious establishments, as well as the feelings of disenchantment towards the social world in which Unity Fellowship Church members live, Archbishop Bean intentionally incorporates therapeutic language into his sermons, and into his church rituals. The aim and consequence of the language of therapy at Unity is to increase members' "psychological capital." Therapy, here, functions as a form of re-education, by equipping the "patient-student"—here, the congregation members—with "psychological capital" and teaching them how to live with life's contradictions.[1]

Reverend Paulette, in fact, identified the main goals of Unity Fellowship Church in psychological terms:

> I mean everything is about, you know, empowering, enlightening, and lifting people up, whether they're positive or negative. Because it all. . . . A lot of it comes back down to the self-esteem issue. If you feel good about yourself and you know that God loves you, no matter what, then you're not going to continue inappropriate behavior. And people who are [HIV] positive can re-infect themselves, can infect themselves with a different strain. They can infect someone who is negative. So . . . if you feel good about yourself, you're going to be careful and not do those behaviors. So, I think everything from the pulpit is trying to empower and lift people up.

Reverend Paulette acknowledged that as an institution, Unity has little control over homophobia and other prejudices. What Unity does try to do in response to these prejudices is to simply help congregation members "understand that they are whole and complete, just exactly as they are." The hope, of course, is that "the more we work with them and the more that they get

123

that they're fine [and that] there's nothing wrong with them," congregation members' perceptions of themselves will begin to improve.

Minister Pepper confirmed the necessity of a therapeutically driven church culture. She noted:

> I was forty-years-old when I first heard "God loves you exactly as you are." And once I started to say that to people in the community when I facilitated workshops or whatever, I could tell that they had never heard it before either. . . . [I]t really does need to be said, you know? Because as a generation of people who have been oppressed, people who are less than, who have little, who have no education in some cases, you know, who are not doing as well as others, we need to hear, "You are perfect in every way. You're exactly how you're supposed to be." Because in our community, one of our main focus is on trying to be like somebody else. We have people who everything that we do is fashion and after someone else. Hairstyles, nails, whatever. And we're trying. . . . We tried so often to make ourselves into somebody else.

Because many of the congregation members at Unity Fellowship Church have experienced trauma in their lives, it makes sense that the language at Unity is distinctly therapeutically oriented. Indeed, even the church founder and pastor likens his church to a hospital, suggesting that for church members, there is a need to cure or heal, or at least a need for therapeutic language. Therapeutic language, thus, is a shared language at Unity Fellowship Church. Even if trauma and oppression do not accurately describe the experiences of all congregation members at Unity, the point is that, at Unity Fellowship Church, the therapeutic language is shared. This shared language is a common reference point for congregation members, even if not all congregation members adhere to it or benefit from it.[2]

The therapeutic language at Unity serves at least two purposes. First, against the disenchantment of the world, Archbishop Bean proposes therapy, with a major goal being to help congregation members help themselves. His aim is to re-socialize congregation members with respect to what it means to be religious, gay, and marginalized. This re-socialization process, however, demands a highly expressive-individualistic language that is psychologically beneficial to the person.

Second, Unity Fellowship Church members' GLBT identity, in particular, has forced them to question the relevance of prior religious scripts. For congregation members at Unity, the established strategies of action that characterize traditional religion and traditional religious organizations are neither relevant nor effective. As a result, they were forced to seek out new symbolic resources, and even a new religious setting, to anchor and reconstruct themselves and their self-identities. These reasons are why Unity Fellowship Church members have affiliated themselves with, and fellowship at, Unity Fellowship Church.

Unity Fellowship Church members desperately seek freedom. Foremost, they seek freedom from oppressive religion and oppressive religious organizations, but also freedom from the pain associated with marginalization and trauma. Other times, freedom sometimes means simply being left alone by others or not having other people's values, ideas, or styles of life imposed upon them. This often refers to the desire to be independent of the ideologies, constraints, and impositions of dominant society. Still, other times, freedom refers to "the right to the means for achieving inclusion."[3] This latter form of freedom is a collective goal that seeks to gain the privileges of full membership or citizenship, or attainment of political (or religious) independence or rights. At Unity, this translates to mean liberation from sexual oppression and social equality for GLBT people.

The function of therapeutic language is to enable some of these freedoms. Notably, at Unity Fellowship Church the clergy often specify acts of pain that cause inner turmoil, and offer expressive remedies in response. Commonly, the clergy encourage the disclosure of secrets or disclosure of past traumas. Implied here is that talking about one's pain is therapeutic, lending to healing and psychological liberation.

For more collectivist goals, the clergy at Unity blend therapeutic language with a social-justice language. Most commonly, Archbishop Bean combats the perceptions of GLBT people as aberrant by framing homosexuality as not freely chosen. Homosexuality is said to be biologically determined and even God-given; therefore, homosexuality is not only natural and normal but divinely inspired. But because GLBT status is said to be ascribed at birth, rather than freely chosen, GLBT people are therefore considered a minority group. The minority status then allows GLBT people to claim unjustified discrimination at the hands of religious organizations, clergy, and others who have espoused homophobic viewpoints. The solution, then, becomes one of according the same rights and protections to homosexuals as those granted to other minority groups in America.[4, 5]

The therapeutic language that characterizes Unity Fellowship Church necessarily involves emotions and feelings. Therapeutic societies, of course, place primacy on feelings and emotional expressions, both affectively and verbally. On the one hand, because the "truth" of feelings cannot be verified, and because so many factors make feelings (and arguments based on feelings) seem irrational, or at least elusive, one cannot rely on simply feelings as representative of "truth."[6] This is particularly the case when they are used to demand large-scale social changes.

On the other hand, pain or trauma is especially representative of human truth, according to Dawne Moon, because "pain seems to be something you can only know when you feel it; it isn't open to outside interpretation. Pain seems natural, yet it is something Christians are called to revere (for example, Christ on the cross) and to alleviate."[7] The "language of pain" therefore is appealing for practicing Christians, because pain is a vital component of Christian teachings, often linked to the teachings and life of Jesus Christ, the "suffering servant."[8] Moon further argues:

> To harm another is wrong . . . but to feel pain can be almost sacred. Because of the truth value of pain and because members idealized the church's role of showing compassion to the needy and giving relief to those in need, pro-gay church members could think and speak of gay people's pain as the reason the church must be open to them. Seeing God as a universal redeemer and sustainer, they could see pain as the opposite of God's intent.[9]

The language of pain, hence, demands that people respond with compassion, necessitating a counter-language of therapy. The goal of the therapeutic language is two-fold. First, therapeutic language is used to negotiate the terms under which GLBT worshippers and other marginalized individuals are brought into the church. That is, it provides a reason why people *need* to be in church, presumably a space of healing. Second, the therapeutic language is used to facilitate healing among congregation members who are suffering, whether from external or internal forces.

As beneficial as therapeutic religion might be to the traumatized and marginalized, the attention to therapy in a religious organization may have unintended consequences. This was illustrated at Unity Fellowship Church. There is no question that Unity Fellowship Church is a "messy" church in many ways. It is messy in that the underbelly of the congregation, and of congregation members, are exposed. The congregants' sexual orientation, sexuality, and even sexual habits are on open display, transgressions and illicit activities are disclosed, and highly traumatic pasts are uncovered. In general, congregation members' unconventional behaviors (i.e., overt sexual expressions), bumps, bruises, and scars are made known at Unity, even when no specific persons are singled out or called to task.

Archbishop Bean himself is far from perfect. He is a flawed man, just like his flock, but he is a compassionate man. This is what draws people to him, and this is what, in particular, draws the least of them to him, and him to them. That is to say, in spite of some congregation members' critiques of what they perceived were excess freedoms at Unity Fellowship Church, and congregation members' behavioral excesses, the reason they remain at Unity is that, in spite of the perceived messiness of their church, their church—and especially the church founder and pastor—accepts them as they are.

Thus, what makes Unity Fellowship Church so unique is this: This congregation is symbolic of compassion and acceptance, particularly towards those with non-normative statuses. It is a space for society's throwaways to worship and fellowship with few constraints. It is a vital religious community in which members share a world of suffering. This community is compassionate towards people with non-normative statuses and histories, because this religious community is a community with a shared history of human suffering. The question then becomes not how to avoid, eliminate, or justify suffering, but how to respond appropriately to it.

Unity Fellowship Church reminds us that therapeutic religion is a viable option for the marginalized, disenfranchised, and other people needing healing. Therapeutic religion is important because it does not deny life but rather enhances it.[10] As the respondents in this study confirm, Unity Fellowship Church, in one way or another, has contributed to the betterment of human life.

This is not to suggest, however, that Unity Fellowship Church and churches with a distinctly therapeutic orientation are end-all cures for either individual or societal maladies. Nor is therapy a replacement for religion. Indeed, in spite of the infusion of therapy in the religious messages and rituals, the therapeutic culture has not displaced the religious order at Unity Fellowship Church. The point is that Unity is only one of many options that may help worshippers to organize and enhance their own lives. Therapeutic-religious societies such as Unity Fellowship Church mix therapy and religion in relatively equal doses, and teach their members how to reduce their own suffering by coming to terms with who they are, rather than what society wants them to be. In all, such communities strive to help their members cope with life's contradictions.

Perhaps more than anything, Unity Fellowship Church—symbolized here by its founder and pastor, Archbishop Bean—inspires hope. Archbishop Bean understands that sometimes the conditions of people's lives do not inspire much care or hope, either for themselves or for others. Archbishop Bean, accordingly, not only affirms congregation members' experiences, but he promises them a better life. He provides an innovative church life that enhances congregation members' worship experience. He inspires them to become healthier, more productive, and more civically minded people. In establishing the Unity Fellowship Church community, he also encourages participants to forge lasting and supportive relationships with each other. In all, Archbishop Bean, through a distinctly therapeutic vocabulary, provides the interpretive resources necessary for congregation members to lead healthier, more productive, and more engaged lives.

Archbishop Bean is a therapist to his congregant-patients in many respects. He draws from many of the elements that Sigmund Freud, the father of psychoanalysis, originated. He underscores the role of introspection and self-discovery, and emphasizes therapy, primarily in the expressive sense. In the end, though, Archbishop Bean departs from Freud in two significant ways. First, Archbishop Bean is foremost a pastor, not a psychoanalyst or therapist. Second, and even more significant, for Freud, love is not a final solution but merely a therapeutic one.[11] For Archbishop Bean, in contrast, love is religious, therapeutic, *and* the ultimate solution.

CONCLUSION

This case study gives some texture to how marginalized persons respond to, and mediate, oppression, by engaging in the tools with which their religious community has empowered them. In this case, the tools are heavily therapeutic; they give people permission to engage in self-expressions and emotional release, and they strive to affirm the total person, regardless of the person's social identities and background.

This study also finds that the experimental nature of therapeutic societies may contribute to excesses and an appearance of "messiness." In this study, the therapeutic ethic that characterizes Unity Fellowship Church has led to some freedoms that are normally disallowed in the congregational setting. These new-found freedoms have resulted in certain overt behaviors, practices, and utterances. These behaviors, while giving the impression of "messiness," really represent deviations from conventional, if not rigid, religious and congregational norms. More specifically, what may appear to church outsiders (and even to some church insiders) as "messy" at Unity Fellowship Church actually represents a resistance, if not unwillingness, by the church leader and his congregants to be stifled, suppressed, socially controlled, and dehumanized.

The aforementioned outcomes, while representing deviations from conventional religious and congregational norms, do not imply that therapeutic societies simply disregard conventional norms altogether. Indeed, the interview narratives and analysis of the sermons in this study suggest that congregation members desire rules, boundaries, and traditions, even while embracing new freedoms.

Moreover, for the people the therapeutic societies serve, the occasional "messiness" that may arise matters far less than the need for diverse functions that blend both religion and therapy. This is particularly the case if the immediate goal of the congregation or society is to eliminate human suffering, in which case distinctly therapeutic and highly experimental ways of doing things may be pivotal in helping to reintegrate the wounded back into the community folds.

NOTES

1. Rieff, *Triumph of the Therapeutic.*
2. Eliasoph and Lichterman, "Culture in Interaction," 743.
3. Williams, "Constructing the Public Good," 133.
4. Melinda S. Miceli, "Morality Politics vs. Identity Politics: Framing Processes and Competition among Christian Right and Gay Social Movement Organizations," *Sociological Forum* 20, no. 4 (2005): 602.
5. Unfortunately, such collectivist goals are far-reaching, for therapeutic language espoused in a single congregation alone is insufficient to effectuate this large-scale change.
6. Moon, *God, Sex, and Politics,* 182.
7. Ibid., 225.
8. Ibid., 222.
9. Ibid., 225.
10. Betsworth, *Social Ethics,* 93.
11. Rieff, *Triumph of the Therapeutic,* 377.

Appendix

Methodological Challenges

FIELD ENTRY

January 20, 2002, was the first time I visited Unity Fellowship Church, located in South Los Angeles, California. I initially had difficulty locating this church, for I was expecting the traditional physical image of a church (e.g., an imposing stone building with a steeple). The church, however, was situated in an industrial block, although most of the businesses in the area, including a dental clinic, were now abandoned. The church itself was located in what appears to be a former warehouse. It was a pinkish concrete building with no windows whatsoever. The entry door was buttressed by a wrought iron door.

Minority AIDS Project (MAP) was located directly across the street from the church, although there is no direct reference to HIV or AIDS; there is simply a very unassuming MAP logo. A sign at the entryway of the church building, in contrast, proclaimed that "God is Love and Love is for Everyone." This, as I later discovered, was the church motto.

One of the first things that struck me was the conspicuous absence of visual religious symbols at Unity Fellowship Church, with the exception of small crosses and candles in the worship area. Nowhere on the exterior of the church building, a converted warehouse, were religious symbols evident. Also absent were pictorial or sculptural depictions of Jesus Christ or any other religious figures. This absence, I later discovered, was intentional. First, it served to not alienate visitors from other faith traditions, by permitting them to draw from non-Protestant or even non-Christian sources for inspiration and strength. Second, it did not impose on congregants any fixed images of, say, Jesus Christ (e.g., a white Jesus, a white God, etc.). The absence of religious symbols at Unity Fellowship Church then, was consistent with the general fluid and expansive nature of this church's religion.

When I entered Unity Fellowship Church for the first time, a young African-American man with dreadlocks who was perhaps in his late 20s or early 30s greeted me very warmly. He wore a burgundy dress shirt and black pants and shoes. I was unsure of his role at the church and wondered if he might be an official church representative or a greeter of some sort. He welcomed me and informed me when services would begin.

As I waited for worship service to start, I studied the artwork and the photos in the church lobby. I was quite surprised by how sparse the interior was. In one corner was a glass display of photos of the founding member of Minority AIDS Project, the Reverend Carl Bean (now archbishop), who is currently the C.E.O. of MAP. There are many plaques that Reverend Bean received in appreciation of his community work. There were also photos of a younger, thinner Carl Bean, often with the warm, beaming smile that endeared him to congregation members and strangers alike.

On the wall near the single desk in the lobby were photos of the church clergy. There was a medium-sized fish tank in the lobby, along with a few African-themed artwork on the walls. There were no other furnishings. The lobby contained three doors: the entry door, a second door that led to the worship space, and a third door that led to the community area. I peeked into the community area and was surprised by how empty it was. It was essentially one very large, gym-like room with a small stage area and little else.

The church spokesperson who greeted me informed me that there were fifteen churches across the nation affiliated with Unity Fellowship Church. He also notified me that the church founder, Carl Bean, no longer presided over Sunday services, because he was currently on the east coast. As it turned out, Archbishop Bean was away from the mother church, visiting the fifteen daughter churches at the time.

I was under the impression that the church had services every hour, so I arrived around 10:30 a.m. I discovered that I was misinformed and that church service started at 11:30 a.m. Since I had arrived early, I was able to observe the testimonial service that preceded Sunday worship service. Initially, I was hesitant about observing testimonial service, as I thought it was a private service for only those who had testimonies, but the church spokesperson encouraged me to attend, and so I did. I found this particular part of Sunday service to be one of the most distinctive and most profound features of the church.

As soon as I entered the sanctuary for testimonial service, I felt this church was not very "church-like" in decor. First of all, I was shocked to see musical instruments more appropriate for a rock concert—a candy apple red drum set and electric guitars. There also was a grand piano, but, to my surprise, no organ. My expectations obviously were very antiquated, based on a very traditional and very unidimensional church image.

Instead of pews, the worship area contained rows and rows of interlocking pink-cushioned seats. The worship space was quite sparse in decor. There was a rainbow-colored African tapestry and a framed piece of watercolor that says "God is Love," but other than that, there was little else. There were no stained glass windows. In fact, there were no windows period, which made the service area quite dark. I wondered to myself how people would exit the sanctuary in the event of an emergency.

There were three or four individuals in the front of the service area, near the pulpit, and all of them were African-American men. I did not want to intrude, so I sat toward the middle of the worship area, near the end of one of the rows of seats. I vaguely overheard the conversation between the three gentlemen in the front of the room. Two of the men looked perfectly healthy, and a third looked somewhat gaunt; indeed, his face appeared skeletal. The latter person informed the other two attendees that his doctor had put him on a regimented diet of salad. His statement was an acute reminder to me that some of the congregation members were, indeed, HIV-positive.

Only a handful of people attended the testimonial service. A junior clergy walked in and then walked up and down the service area, but concentrated near the area that was most heavily populated. He asked if anyone would like to provide their testimony. Each person who testified greeted the congregation with statements along the lines of, "Good morning, Unity."

Slowly, people trickled in. I counted seventeen in attendance, all African American. The man whom I had previously overheard tells other members that he was on a regimen of salad testified how grateful he was to be alive. He disclosed his medication, noting that he took three pills per day. Another individual indicated that he sometimes could barely get up in the morning, but was grateful that he could. He knew that, in spite of his condition, he has it better off than other people.

Two women entered the service area, both dressed impeccably in a style reminiscent of the 1980s Dynasty-era extravagance. One appeared to be a white woman, and her companion was an extremely skeletal and frail African-American woman who wore a black dress and black hat with a quarter veil. The latter gave her testimony. She indicated that she had lost her hair (which I didn't notice when she entered, as it was hidden by her hat). She confessed that her friend had dressed her up so she could look presentable in church. The woman was very thin and was clearly ill. The woman said that sometimes she had difficulty getting up in the morning, but she, too, was grateful that she was able to get up and was grateful for what she did have.

A heavyset woman who wore a rather tight, low-cut red dress, and had extremely long, curly, press-on nails, loudly announced her difficulties at work. She said that she had been promoted but that her boss was essentially "a bitch." Her use of profanities surprised me, but yet I was secretly pleased by the openness of the forum. In testimonial services, men and women openly described experiences and lives characterized by deprivation, ailing health, relationship fractures, drug use, among other difficulties. I marveled at how forthcoming these testimonials were. What struck me, above all, was the candor of the testimonials. It suggested to me that Unity Fellowship Church was not a run-of-the-mill church. Indeed, many of the interview respondents in this study described the churches they previously attended as being too rules-oriented and too restricted, to the point that congregation members were forced to restrain themselves verbally and affectively. Their churches seemed to silence them.

The first worship service I attended at Unity Fellowship Church began at 11:30 a.m. The worship area filled quickly. The congregation was overwhelmingly African American, with an equal mix of men and women. There were approximately five white individuals, and maybe two or three Latinos were present. I was the single Asian in attendance.

Also prominent was the proportion of the congregation who appeared to be ailing. While most of the attendees appeared physically healthy, there were a few that looked quite ill. A few people looked quite emaciated, and I suspected that they had experienced bodily wasting, given their gaunt, skeletal appearance. In light of the fact that Unity Fellowship Church is an AIDS ministry, and linked to the Minority AIDS Project, I suspected that some of the congregation members might be at the end stages of HIV disease, AIDS, and were terminally ill.

The HIV/AIDS focus was even more apparent when the minister presiding over the testimonial service discussed the high rates of HIV among African Americans. The minister stressed the need to continue educating people about HIV/AIDS, and also encouraged people to openly talk about HIV with their friends. The minister expressed gratitude for both Unity Fellowship Church and Minority AIDS Project, where he works.

The morning service began with a processional, in which the church choir and clergy marched in singing "Walk in the Light." The clergy entered in ascending order by rank, with the presiding pastor entering last. There was live music throughout the service, and a small multi-racial choir (predominantly African American, but there was a white woman) sang and danced along with the music. The service was characterized by high audience participation in the form of dancing, clapping, singing, arm-waving, and bursts of affirmation. The acoustics were remarkable, at least early on in the field work. Because the service area is relatively small and compact, with a low ceiling (consisting of wood beams), the audience was able to literally feel the amplified music. The ground seemed to vibrate with the music.

When I began my study, a female clergy was presiding over the congregation while Archbishop Bean was away touring the daughter churches. This particular clergy added elements and rituals to the church services that apparently agitated some congregation members, because once Archbishop Bean returned, these rituals were eliminated. This included a morning prayer that began with the dimming of the lights, a low, dull, drumbeat, and the clergy "calling the ancestors." At first, I was a bit puzzled, if not slightly concerned, by this ritual, because I did not know what to expect in the darkened room. The acoustics of the room seemed to amplify the drumming and the occasionally high-pitched yells and squeals, lending to an otherworldly feel. I also was initially perplexed as to why the service involved a ritual that appeared more Native American than African, but concluded that although this congregation was primarily African American, it really was a multicultural congregation, and this was evident by the fact that the presiding clergy at the time incorporated aspects of other cultures.

The entire ambience from this particular ritual—from the dimmed lights to the constant, low drumbeat, to the amplified acoustics—produced a meditative-like feeling for me, but perhaps that was because I was new to the environment and my senses were hyper-alert. As one congregation member, Wanda, described it, this ritual "took you on a spiritual plane."

Prayers and announcements followed this ritual. A junior clergy provided details with respect to community events that involved HIV/AIDS. The clergy also provided a prayer list. During this portion of the service, the lights were once again dimmed, and the clergy recited a list of ailing congregation members, and requested that the church keep these members in their thoughts and prayers.

One portion of the service that I did not at all expect was a ritual known as "hug and love." In this ritual, congregation members were instructed to walk around the worship area, greeting attendees, embracing them, and affirming their presence with a verbal "You are very special." As a somewhat shy person, and a person new to this church setting, the physicality of this ritual made me a bit uncomfortable. I am not an outwardly affectionate person, so it was not my style to randomly approach strangers, hug them, and provide verbal affirmations of them.

Nonetheless, I sensed that this ritual was a pivotal part of the church culture. The verbal affirmations and the physical affirmation (hugging) evoked profound emotions for some of the attendees. In fact, it was this ritual that many of the interview respondents cited as particularly memorable with their first visit to the church. Some of the respondents recalled being moved to tears when congregation members—strangers at the time—approached them and embraced them. For some of the respondents, the hugging seemed to indicate an emotional and social connection, but also an unspoken but shared understanding of whatever it was that the huggee was going through at the time.

Other embodied aspects of Unity's religious culture also proved to be a source for my initial discomfort during my field entry. I observed how physically involved worship service was at Unity. As someone who is completely unrhythmic, as well as introverted and restrained, I refrained from dancing or singing along with the music. As the choir sang, congregation members and visitors around me stood up, clapped, danced, and sang out loud, yelled, and cried. A few congregation members beat or shook their tambourines loudly and enthusiastically.

A three-year-old girl, the granddaughter of one of the congregation members, sat in front of me during the first service I attended on January 20, 2002. She occasionally glanced back at me. At one point, she motioned with her hands for me to get up and dance, like the others. I finally got up and clapped my hands along to the musical beat, but I refrained from other bodily movements. At another service, during one of the musical numbers, a number of church attendees rose to their feet, with one or both arms outstretched. The gentleman behind me gently prodded me to stand. He took my hand gently, and stretched my arm, and stated to me, "Ain't nothing wrong with praising the lord." As my field work progressed, and I became more and more familiar with the congregation and the church members, and became more accustomed to the worship rituals, I became far more responsive to the music, in particular, although I never did exhibit the level of physicality that some congregation members displayed during service. The embodied response to music was one I could adapt to without much discomfort, unlike the hug-and-love portion of service.

However, there was one element that continually made me uncomfortable, and that was the physicality of some of the congregation members. While I welcomed the congregants' warmth and affection toward me, on a few occasions congregation members displayed extremely inappropriate behaviors. Some of these might have been unintentional violations of my personal and physical space, but other behaviors were outright inappropriate. At the conclusion of one worship service, for example, a female congregation member and I greeted each other. Her greeting, however, was far more than I anticipated. The woman leaned down to hug me and, as she was doing so, gave me a big, long, wet, sloppy kiss on my neck that left a trail of saliva on me. This behavior shocked me and, frankly, left me a bit startled and angry. At another service, during the affirmation ritual, the same woman approached me and forcefully pressed her chest into mine as she embraced me. A month later, the same woman greeted me during affirmation, and just as she had done before, hugged me really hard, too hard, literally crushing me into her chest. There were other instances of "inappropriate hugs."

During the affirmation ritual of Bible study one night, one woman—a complete stranger—embraced me from behind and kissed me soundly on the cheek, and then kissed me passionately on the neck, which completely startled me. Another congregation member, to whom I was more familiar, also kissed me quite passionately when I had a cold, and declared that, "I'm not afraid of your cold." It should be noted that the latter congregation member has a habit of wavering between affection and anger. When she greeted people, she was unusually "affectionate" and had a habit of kissing them. At one Friday night street ministry, I decided that I would let it be known that I wish not to be kissed by her any longer. Another participant at the street ministry (a male), however, beat me to it; he declared that night to the woman that he did not care for her affections. When the congregation member attempted to kiss him, he explicitly articulated his dislike of people kissing him.

It should be noted that the above behaviors are not necessarily indicative of the culture at Unity Fellowship Church. Not all the congregation members behave inappropriately. In fact, most congregation members do not behave inappropriately. I also did not think that these instances of inappropriate physical behaviors necessarily represented certain congregation members' romantic interest in me. These were more likely idiosyncrasies on the part of the individuals, or else they stemmed from severe mental illnesses. Both the clergy and non-clergy interview respondents, in fact, have noted the prevalence of mental illness in the congregation. It was disclosed to me that the woman at the street outreach with a habit of kissing people had serious mental-health issues. When she was on her medications, she was friendly and affectionate; when she was off her meds, she became unusually moody and angry and verbally would lash out at people.

All in all, the worship service at Unity Fellowship Church could not have been more different than what I had anticipated. There was a carnival feel to the worship service, attributed to the assorted colors and ostentatious displays of fashion and make-up, the highly emotive dances, and the emotional outpourings in response to sermons and worship music. The congregation members also seemed genuinely warm and friendly, which was not at all what I had expected; I had expected aloofness, distance, and suspicion of my presence. Instead, congregation members who were complete strangers welcomed me and embraced me, and in the years since I first visited Unity, the congregation members continued to display their warmth and affection toward me.

My first visit at Unity Fellowship Church moved me. The experience felt so otherworldly, temporarily transforming me to an environment to which I was unfamiliar. In addition to the carnival nature of the worship service, there was a warmth to the environment. Everyone seemed so happy and friendly, and genuinely so, a marked contrast to real life. The contrast was so striking that I could not help but feel somewhat dejected after I left the church premises after my first visit.

My encounters with gravely ill people who likely were suffering from the end stages of AIDS also contributed to my dejection. Some of the people in attendance could barely deal with the physical effects of the disease, and at least one could barely walk. Yet, I marveled at how they still managed to make it to church. My spirits were buoyed somewhat in that I sensed from the start that Unity Fellowship Church seemed to be a place where people affected by HIV/AIDS could go, where they would not be judged and would be welcomed by all, embraced by all—physically and emotionally. It was a place where people could openly express their frustrations yet simultaneously find good in those experiences.

NEGOTIATING THE FIELD AS AN OUTSIDER

Fieldworkers' social characteristics fundamentally shape the kinds of interactions and relations that develop from the field setting and, hence, the character and degree of immersion in the field.[1] In this study, particularly relevant attributes include my status as a researcher, my religious inexperience, my race/ethnicity, and my sexual orientation. These attributes shaped the way the research subjects defined, evaluated, and responded to me, but they also shaped how I interpreted what I saw in the field.

Outing Myself as a Researcher

I introduced myself to the clergy at Unity Fellowship Church early on, and made my research intentions clear. I communicated most often with a clergy who functioned as the church administrator. I slowly introduced myself to congregation members, particularly as my attendance became more regular and members became more familiar with me. When it became clear that I intended to focus my study on this particular congregation, I set up a face-to-face meeting with Archbishop Carl Bean, the church founder and pastor, to inform him of my research intentions and to secure his permission for the study.

I realized that I had to reveal my status as a researcher to congregation members early in my field work, in order to avoid deception and to prevent any misconceptions, but also because my racially discordant status made the disclosure inevitable. In other instances, issues related to sexual orientation forced the disclosure.

Early in my field work, one congregation member introduced herself to me. It turned out that the congregation member was interested in me in a non-platonic way, because she quickly asked if I were gay. At that point, I revealed to her my researcher status and briefed her about my project. The congregation member appeared a bit cautious then, and asked what my plans were in terms of the research. I indicated that, at the time, it was my intention to produce a paper for a graduate class, but that I also had hoped to base my dissertation from data collected at this church. I gave this congregant my contact information and indicated that I would eventually like to interview her, or any other church members, to see how they view the church, whether the church has helped them, whether they have attended other churches, and so forth.

The congregation member again articulated her suspicion and informed me that a lot of researchers come into the church setting and simply form their own judgments. This was particularly true of white researchers. She explicitly verbalized her suspicion of researchers—especially white researchers—noting that she is very much aware that outsiders impose their own views and unfairly judge the setting, culture, and people to which they are not familiar.

My researcher status was brought to attention more than two years later, in June of 2004, when I attended Spiritual Renewal, a religious program that was held weekly, on a weekday evening. Two congregation members, a couple, were not aware that I was conducting research on their church until a church clergy had pointed out my researcher status during the spiritual renewal class. One of the women asked me in what context I was interested in the church. She inquired whether I was focusing on black gays in particular, a valid question considering that I was not black. But her question highlighted not only my outsider status as a racialized "other," but also my outsider status as a researcher, rather than community member. Moreover, her inquiry reminded me that African-American individuals are all too aware of outsiders entering their community and studying them, and potentially misinterpreting their cultures.

I responded to the congregation member's query with a statement along the lines that I was interested in Unity Fellowship Church because I had heard that this church was a forerunner in terms of certain health care issues—notably, in terms of HIV/AIDS. This was not an untruth, for when I embarked on the study, I had every intention of focusing on the HIV dimension of the church; indeed, a key reason why I selected Unity Fellowship Church as the site of analysis was that it was an AIDS ministry. However, I also selected this church because it was predominantly African American, and I felt that religious organizations, in general, potentially could play a leading role in the battle against HIV/AIDS, which has devastated the African-American population.

Hence, while my response was not entirely untrue, it was clear that I had to withhold some information. This is a methodological and ethical challenge in the field. As Emerson suggested, field work often involves "secret-keeping," wherein the fieldworkers restrict the information they provide with respect to the research focus.[2] Thorne noted that fieldworkers often provide self-introductions that are "partial truths." These "partial truths" are often intentionally vague, and even misleading, as to the identity and purpose of the research.[3] Similarly, Fine noted that some ethnographers intentionally sugarcoat their introductions to research subjects, whose cooperation they must obtain.[4]

Aware of congregation members' suspicions of researchers, I tried to establish rapport first with congregation members, by spending considerable time at the church. I paid attention to the dynamics between researcher and research subjects and recognized that my race/ethnicity, social class, gender, and sexual orientation potentially may influence the research subjects' responses and interactions with me. As I attended worship services regularly, congregation members became more familiar with me and more comfortable with my presence. I also participated in a number of church groups and events—notably, a street ministry that met weekly, on Friday night, in the Skid Row area of downtown Los Angeles.

As an outsider, I needed someone to assist in gaining entry into the community. In some cases, entry into a church group was facilitated by a clergy or by a congregation member with whom I had at least friendly acquaintance. For instance, when I attended a transgender leadership council, one female clergy in attendance introduced me to the group and "put in a good word" for me, and about me, after I introduced myself to the group and briefed them on my study. The clergy explained that I had participated in her women's support group and was an "integral" part of that group. Having been legitimized by a clergy provided some legitimacy among the group of transgender individuals to whom I was not entirely familiar.

A few congregation members generously offered assistance. At the conclusion of his interview, for instance, Samuel inquired whether I had any questions for him with respect to the church and church culture. I suspected that he felt that as an outsider in the community, I might not fully understand some of the aspects of life at Unity, particularly the religious life of African-American men and women, as well as the religious life of GLBT people. Samuel, of course, was correct in this assumption. Selma, an active participant of church life, provided words of wisdom when I interviewed her, although her advice was not directly at me exclusively. She stated:

> [I]f you really don't understand. . . . If your field is working with people with HIV or AIDS or gay people, whatever, or African-American, and you're Chinese and whatever, you go in there and you have to learn that culture. You may not agree with everything that goes on, but you have to show compassion, because you don't show compassion, then you're not being of service. So it's like each time that I come in here [to church], I have to show compassion, because I want to be of service . . .

Spending time with congregation members both in church and outside of church facilitated a greater understanding of the church culture and minimized the artificiality that often exists in relationships between researchers and subjects. As congregation members became more familiar with me, they also exhibited more comfort around me and were willing to be more forthcoming. In fact, by the time I conducted the face-to-face interviews, a number of the respondents appeared to express their beliefs and worldviews in an uninhibited manner. At times, congregation members even used the interview time as almost a therapy session. A few interview respondents, for instance, became teary when discussing their history and transformations at Unity Fellowship Church, while a few respondents expressed frustration with some of the church affairs and interactions.

The Religious Outsider

The fact that I was the sole Asian person in attendance did not bother me in the least bit. Nor did the fact that around me were flamboyantly gay men, women, and transgendered people, as well as the not-so-flamboyant ones. I was drawn to both racial/ethnic and sexual minorities. Whatever discomfort I might have had at the first or subsequent visit to Unity Fellowship Church had more to do with my own religious inexperience, which was quite conspicuous at the earlier visits. At my first visit, a three-year-old-girl, the granddaughter of one of the congregation members, noticed how wooden I looked. With her grandmother's encouragement, the little girl led me to the front of the pulpit area, where she lit a candle and motioned for me to do the same.

I observed a disruption during another worship service—or at least what I thought was disruption. A man was yelling and moving down the aisle that separated the seating areas. I could not see his precise movements, because my view was obstructed, but I did notice quick, jerking movements and thought he was flopping around on the floor like a fish out of water. I observed that looks of concern on the religious leaders' faces, which in turn caused me to become concerned. At one point, I assumed the man had collapsed, because he was no longer visible. Perhaps he was having a seizure; yet I wondered why no one came to his aid. Initially I was a bit puzzled, then annoyed, even slightly angry, that a church that claimed to be welcoming and opening to all would sit by so callously and not help a man who potentially had a life-threatening medical condition. I contemplated calling 9-1-1, but ultimately resisted. Since I was new to this church community, and since no one was helping the man, I concluded that his "condition" did not warrant serious attention. After all, it could not be possible that all the congregation members—and notably the clergy—would be so heartless as to not come to the aid of one of their own. And because no one was assisting him, I likely was misinterpreting the event. Given the ambiguity of the situation, and unsure of the correct response, I relied on the behaviors of those around me as cues for social action (or, in this case, non-action). I ultimately determined that the man likely was having some sort of religious transformation, albeit a violent one.

At the conclusion of this service, I asked a woman who was sitting one seat to the left of me about the disruption. I apologized to this woman for my religious ignorance, but expressed my concern for the man with the "seizure." I told her that I would not have been so concerned myself, but became concerned because the clergy looked concerned themselves. I mentioned that I felt it was possible that the man was having a religious transformation, but that I was not sure and thought that perhaps he had physically collapsed. I asked her if he was okay. The woman chuckled and said that he was having a religious experience. The fact that the woman was chuckling hinted to my naivety—specifically, my inability to discern between a medical condition and a religious transformation, albeit one that was a bit theatrical.

There were other instances in which I looked to congregation members for cues on how to behave. After one service, congregation members lined up to greet and "bless" a particular clergy, who was about to start seminary classes. I observed that the congregation members who met with this clergy each gave her a warm embrace and/or a kiss. Many placed money in her hands. I asked one congregation member about the cash gifts and was a bit embarrassed, indicating that I did not realize we were supposed to give money, as I seldom carry cash with me. The congregation member insisted that we were not required to give cash, but that sometimes our words are enough.

On a few occasions, I was forced to reveal my religious non-affiliation. During a commute together to a Friday-night community service with the church, Deacon Pepper (now minister) briefly inquired about my religious affiliation during the course of our conversation. I told her that I did not have a religious affiliation, and that I did not grow up with religion. She seemed unphased by this revelation.

Curiously, it was not at church where my non-religiousness became an issue; my non-religiousness became an issue at times at the Friday night street ministry. This ministry included a small group of volunteers from the church who either purchased food out of pocket or obtained free food from local food banks. Some of them would cook homemade meals for the homeless. On those nights, Deacon Pepper, usually with a few volunteers, would pick up donations of clothes and shoes from the church, and she and the volunteers would transport the items to the homeless men and women.

There were religious rituals incorporated into the street ministry. Before the street ministry group served dinner to the homeless, for instance, Deacon Pepper would lead a prayer, which usually consisted of praises to God. The ministry also concluded with a circle prayer among the volunteers. During the concluding prayer circle, the volunteers would assemble into a tightly closed circle, with volunteers clutching each other around the waist. Deacon Pepper usually provided a brief prayer, but the prayers were then opened up to all volunteers. The prayers also often included testimonies, with requests that volunteers "pray" for the person providing the testimony. In the prayer circle, I observed that the volunteers often closed their eyes and bowed their heads, so I, too, bowed my head when others provided their prayers and praises. But occasionally I would look up and note that some volunteers were not bowing their heads; some had their eyes opened and were looking at the person speaking. I had assumed the prayer etiquette was to at least bow one's head.

Occasionally, a homeless man or woman would request individual prayers, either during the food service or s/he would join us in the closing prayer circle. One Friday night, a homeless man conversed with me at length and at one point in the conversation requested that I pray for him. I responded, out of naivety, erroneously believing that only ordained people could provide prayers. As a result, I informed the homeless man that I could not pray for him, but that Deacon Pepper could. Later, he asked me why I would not pray for him and seemed slightly annoyed. I indicated that I could not pray for him because I was not religious.

On another night, one rather mischievous homeless man named Nelson had a habit of spouting Bible passages that alluded to the end of the world. He engaged in this behavior a few times, and I observed that some of the homeless people found his behavior rather annoying. Others paid little attention to Nelson. Nelson was a gregarious sort and conversed and pestered the volunteers on occasion. He pointed out to one of the church volunteers that I was the only one who did not respond to him when he spewed out passages from the Bible. Nelson seemed amused by this fact. I indicated to the volunteer that I did not respond to Nelson's end-of-the-world predictions because I was not religious, a point that surprised the volunteer. In fact, he had a stunned looked when I revealed this piece of information. However, he quickly recovered, smiled, and said, "That's okay."

The Racialized "Other"

As the sole Asian person in attendance at services, I became a racialized "other." My status as a racial outsider was conspicuous, even as I became more and more involved with the church. Early in my field work, one congregation member mistook me for a newspaper reporter. The congregation member had seen me at service once before, and just as he did at the first meeting, he greeted me very warmly the second time we encountered. During our second encounter, however, this congregation member inquired where my friends were. I was puzzled and asked what he meant, as I always attended church service alone. The congregation member indicated that he thought I was a newspaper reporter, just as the two people he had observed from months ago were. I suspected he was referring to two Caucasian individuals, one male and one female, who had sat behind me during worship service months ago. Because of my physical proximity to these individuals, and because I was not African American, the congregation member likely assumed I was associated with these two individuals, who turned out to be newspaper reporters. At the prior service, I had borrowed a pen from the Caucasian male, and I observed that the Caucasian woman seated next to him was taking copious notes throughout worship service. I informed the congregation member that I was not associated with these two individuals, and did not know who they were. The congregation member told me they were newspaper reporters from San Diego.

Even when I became more familiar with the congregation and interacted with congregation members on a regular basis, there were inferences to my race/ethnicity. This became especially apparent during the interviews. When I asked Al what he felt was special or unique about his church, he noted the openness and acceptance of the church culture. He stated, as an example, "Just like . . . you know, just like anybody . . . YOU coming here. You know, no one's . . . at least to my knowledge, have looked at you differently [as an Asian], have said, 'What is she doing here?' None of that." Later in the interview, when I inquired about possible reasons for why conflicts erupt at the church, Al stated that conflicts often arise because of "personal issues." Again, he provided an illustration: "Just say, for instance, I had a resentment against women of Asian descent. It has nothing to do with you, but because of me and my own issues and the issues I have unresolved, I take it out on you."

Other interview respondents similarly pointed out my conspicuous racial dissimilarity. This was evident in Reverend Luther's self-definition of "liberation theology," which he associated with concepts of freedom—notably freeing one's mind. In my interview with Reverend Luther, he elaborated as follows:

> Look how big God is. So freeing your mind to know the allness of God is freeing your mind from any barriers. Any barriers. Whether it's your prejudice, whether it's your sexism, whether it's your racism, whether it's your fear. It's removing those barriers. Even if it's for a fleeting moment. To know that God resides in Pam the way God resides in another woman over here. You know, if I only saw you as an Asian woman, then I wouldn't be able to see how the magnificence of this higher power, the creator within you. I wouldn't be able to see that, 'cause I'd be saying, "Oh, no, she's Asian. She doesn't have anything for me. I can't . . ." I just blocked seeing God in you. So freeing your mind says move that out of the way so you can see who this person really

is. So that's freeing your mind to know that allness of that. Freeing your mind, body, and spirit to know the allness of God. Just how big God is, you know? And when you do that, when you free your mind from the fears and all those kinds of things, then when God is present and God is moving, you'll recognize that. You'll say, "That's God moving right there. That's the spirit of God moving in the situation."

I found it particularly interesting that Reverend Luther specifically evoked my status as an Asian woman in his response. He seemed to imply that seeing God in other people meant looking beyond the person's race and ethnicity, particularly if the person's race/ethnicity is discordant with one's own. Yet, by explicitly mentioning racial differences, he is highlighting the fact that I am, in fact, a racialized "other." At the same time, Reverend Luther's point seems to be that seeing God in others means seeing the commonalities and the good in people who may appear different from ourselves. It means overcoming our own prejudices.

Shortly thereafter, when I asked Reverend Luther what the local churches thought about Unity Fellowship Church, and whether Unity has a relationship or partnership with the local churches, Reverend Luther's response became tangential. His response focused on what "being saved" meant. He replied that this particular concept meant death in the metaphysical sense, where people must "die" (or eliminate) their "old, unloving ways." He explained:

See, when I die, the bad stuff . . . and I'm able to now see Pam as a child of God instead of Pam, in my own racist mind, as an Asian woman. When I die to that, that's when the Christ hearts becomes illuminated and God becomes so present. Because I die to my old ways. So I'm born again into my new ways.

In the span of a short timeframe, Reverend Luther had referred to my racial "otherness" at least twice, suggesting that, although I was a familiar face at the predominantly African-American church, I remained a perpetual outsider, particularly in the racial sense. As a racial outsider studying a black community, it was apparent that I did not gain the full trust of some community members, even after more than three years in the field.

In only one instance did I interpret the church interaction as overtly racial. At one worship service, sitting in front of me were two heavyset African-American women. Next to them were three young boys who appeared to be brothers. I assume these boys were the women's sons. All of the boys wore a yellow, sleeveless Spider-man shirt. They appeared to be ages four to seven. The two older boys initially kept staring at me. The older boy, at one point, lifted the outer corner of his eyes, trying to mimic Asians' eye shape. He also stretched out his arms and arranged his arms and hands in a position that is clearly suppose to evoke the stance of a martial-arts position. Although I realized that the boy was young and likely did not understand the racial overtones of his actions, I was nonetheless surprised (I was shocked, actually) and a bit offended. I was rather disappointed by his behavior that I initially felt compelled to either reprimand him or call attention to his behavior to his mother. I was shocked that in this religious setting, given how marginalized everyone was and the many calls to combat racism, that here was an example of a youth who has been taught to engage in racist behaviors. At the same time, I resisted reprimanding the child, or even mentioning the event to his mother, recognizing that I was simply a guest in the setting.

Even Archbishop Bean alluded to my race. When I interviewed Archbishop Bean, we engaged in a dialogue about how God is portrayed. I indicated that James Cone depicted God as exclusively black, because he believed that God needed to represent the oppressed. I observed aloud that Archbishop Bean himself, however, painted God as fluid, as representing anyone and everyone. Archbishop Bean disagreed with Cone's version of a singular black God, explaining, "To me, I don't think you can solve a thing by recreating it with the same thing. I think prejudice is prejudice. I think if that white God was oppressive to me, then your black God is oppressive to you." Shortly thereafter, my Asian-ness was called to attention. This is evident in Archbishop Bean's statement:

> I think we get in trouble when we start getting into tribalism, because what has tribalism ever done but one thing in the end? And so, why can't we, with our enlightenment, seek to move beyond it and not repeat? Because it is repeating. If, in fact, it bruised my ego, my healthiness of self-worth, then why would I want to bruise yours? Why would I say, it looks like me, its eyes are round like mine, not like yours?

By pointing out the differences in eye shape between Asians and non-Asians, Archbishop Bean inadvertently cemented the idea that race was delineated based on perceived physical differences, and that, specifically, to be Asian centered on eye shape primarily.

At a Bible study one evening, Archbishop Bean mentioned to me that he had a watched a documentary on the Discovery Channel that examined young students of color. The hypothesis was that there were genetic differences based on race, which affected intelligence or school achievement somehow. However, contrary to expectations, the study found that the Asian kids were more similar to the black kids, the black kids were similar to the Filipino kids, and so forth. I suggested to Archbishop Bean that society tends to highlight differences in people, but that we're really more similar than we are different. Archbishop Bean concurred.

Most commonly, my presence automatically increased the "diversity" of the setting or group. In fact, on at least three occasions, my presence elicited clergy comments about the diversity of the group. Just before the conclusion of a Spiritual Renewal class, Archbishop Bean remarked about how diverse the participants in this Lent service was, noting, "We have Latinos, Asians, whites, blacks . . . " At another Spiritual Renewal, Reverend Redd commented that there even within this small group of four, the group was "so diverse." He felt it was appropriate that we talk about diversity, about independence, since it was Independence Day weekend. Reverend Redd further indicated that "years and years ago," it would not have been possible to come together in a church setting and have such a diverse group. He stated, "They wouldn't believe it." The racial diversity was again mentioned after two latecomers joined the group. Reverend Redd inquired what the participants believed people would say if we had congregated in a church setting years ago, as people from different ethnicities and cultures. One latecomer echoed Reverend Redd's earlier sentiments, stating that no one would have believed that a group as diverse as ours could come together so peacefully. Hence, it was clear that my presence as an Asian person automatically created diversity, even if I was the sole non-black person there. The mention of "diversity" was explicitly mentioned in my presence multiple times in the course of my study: at the two Spiritual Renewal meetings, at a street outreach one Friday night, at a women's support group, and in the interviews.

Because I was the single Asian person at Unity Fellowship Church, it was expected that some congregation members would be curious about Asians and "Asian-ness." However, the fact that my status as an Asian was evoked so often suggested that, in spite of my growing familiarity in the field, it was evident that I was not considered a full member of the community. At most, I was straddling the line between being a partial insider and a complete outsider; and at other times, I was considered an unwelcome foreigner. This incomplete membership, consequently, likely limited the rapport between some congregation members and myself, and diminished some congregation members' trust in me. But my outsider status seemed to facilitate the trust and rapport of other community members, who seemed very open to discussing church affairs with an outsider, doing so candidly.

A Sexual Minority

Although one's sexual orientation is invisible for the most part, on a few occasions I was forced to disclose my sexual orientation. For the most part, however, I did not disclose my sexual orientation voluntarily, because I did not think my orientation was relevant at the time. Seldom did congregation members explicitly ask about my sexual orientation, but the question was broached. Mostly, though, my sexual orientation went unquestioned. This was likely because Unity Fellowship Church members assumed that I, like they, were gay, as we were all fellowshipping at a gay-centered church. The presumption of "gayness," thus, was expected, given the make-up of this particular church. This assumption became apparent when I interacted with a congregation member and a clergy. The congregation member was describing to me a new program on cable television: *The L-Word*. Although all the characters on this program portray lesbians, the actresses actually were heterosexual, with the exception of one. The congregation member referred to the magazine *LNN*, which featured on its cover a photo of the actresses from *The L-Word*. She pointed out to me which actress was the "real lesbian." Not familiar with this publication, I inquired what the acronym *LNN* stood for. This is the Lesbian News Network.

Later, Reverend Paulette, whom I was meeting, also referred to *LNN* magazine. I mentioned to Reverend Paulette that the congregation member behind the table we were sitting had just informed me about *LNN*, a publication that was available at Minority AIDS Project. The congregation member looked at me in surprise, indicating, "Oh, I just assumed you're a lesbian." I shook my head. Reverend Paulette also seemed surprised, asking me, "You're not a lesbian?" I told them both that I was straight. The congregation member apologized to me, "Pam, I am so sorry for assuming." I insisted there was no need to apologize, because it was understandable that people would assume that I am a lesbian, since the congregation was overwhelmingly GLBT. I informed Reverend Paulette that a couple of the congregation members had actually come out and asked if I were gay. She laughed and said that they were probably "interested." Reverend Paulette and I had a good laugh and noted that the situation here was almost reversed, wherein I had been outed as a straight person at a gay church.

LESSONS FROM THE FIELD

As one would expect, visible differences such as race/ethnicity can make field work especially challenging. This visible social difference can lead to assumptions, suspicion, stereotypes, distrust, and tensions between the researcher and her subjects. As Duneier[5] discovered in his study of African-American book and magazine vendors on the sidewalks of New York City, the outsider status means that the researcher can never know for sure whether s/he has gained the trust of the research subjects. As a result, some of the subjects may distort their responses, and others may give socially desirable responses and responses that they think the researcher wants to hear. The researcher herself may misinterpret the culture and her respondents' statements, because she may not be fully in tune with certain cultural nuances.

The invisible social differences (social class and sexual orientation, for instance), too, can also complicate field work relations, leading to unexpected and even unwanted interactions. In some cases, these exchanges may be particular to specific individuals, indicative of a personality quirk or idiosyncrasy that may not be illustrative of the culture to which the researcher is studying. On the other hand, patterns of these interactions might speak to the particular culture itself—common characteristics among community members, for instance, and/or cultural norms. In the instances in which I experienced "unwanted behavior," for example, I discovered through the interview data that my experiences were not uncommon even among community insiders, who also had experienced untoward behavior. The patterns suggest here that it was not my outsider status that contributed to the unwanted behavior but that the unwanted behaviors were specific to congregation members with mental illnesses.

The tensions I experienced in the field are some common ones that research outsiders face. This is not to say that field work requires an insider status. Indeed, much can be gleaned from a researcher with an outsider status. In this study, my status as a non-member of the church proved advantageous at times. Some of the respondents were very candid with me precisely because I was not a church member. In the privacy of their homes or in other non-church settings where I interviewed them, some of the respondents were forthcoming and quite direct with respect to the going-ons at the church. Had I been a church member, with direct experience and knowledge of the church life and the people who make up the church, the respondents would have been far less forthcoming in their evaluations of their church, their church pastor, and other church members. The tendency for certain research subjects to open up to outsiders was an advantage noted by Ammerman, who stated that outsiders, by virtue of their naiveté, "sometimes provoke a clarity of insight by their very naiveté."[6] However, Ammerman also pointed out that outsiders "may also miss the import of a story or gesture because they do not know enough to 'read between the lines.'"[7]

NOTES

1. Emerson, *Contemporary Field Research*, 116.
2. Ibid., 135.
3. Barrie Thorne, "'You Still Takin' Notes?' Fieldwork and Problems of Informed Consent," *Social Problems* 27, no. 3 (1980): 287.
4. Gary A. Fine, "Ten Lies of Ethnography: Moral Dilemmas in Field Research," *Journal of Contemporary Ethnography* 22 (1993): 275.
5. Mitchell Duneier, *Sidewalk* (New York: Farrar, Straus and Giroux, 1999).
6. Nancy T. Ammerman, "Culture and Identity in the Congregation," in *Studying Congregations: A New Handbook*, eds. Nancy T. Ammerman, Jackson W. Carroll, Carl S. Dudley, and William McKinney (Nashville, TN: Abingdon Press, 1998), 199.
7. Ibid.

References

Ammerman, Nancy T. "Culture and Identity in the Congregation." In *Studying Congregations: A New Handbook*, edited by Nancy T. Ammerman, Jackson W. Carroll, Carl S. Dudley, and William McKinney, 78–104. Nashville, TN: Abingdon Press, 1998.

Andersen, Margaret L. *Thinking about Women: Sociological Perspectives on Sex and Gender,* 5th ed. Boston: Allyn and Bacon, 2000.

Barnes, Sandra L. "Whosoever Will Let Her Come: Social Activism and Gender Inclusivity in the Black Church." *Journal for the Scientific Study of Religion* 45, no. 3 (2006): 371–87.

Becker, Penny Edgell. *Congregations in Conflict: Cultural Models of Local Religious Life.* New York: Cambridge University Press, 1999.

Bellah, Robert N., Richard Madsen, William M. Sullivan, Ann Swidler, and Steven M. Tipton. *Habits of the Heart: Individualism and Commitment in American Life.* Reprint, Berkeley, CA: University of California Press, [1985] 1996.

Berger, Peter L. *The Sacred Canopy: Elements of a Sociological Theory of Religion.* New York: Anchor Books, 1969.

Betsworth, Roger G. *Social Ethics: An Examination of American Moral Traditions.* Louisville, KY: Westminster/John Knox Press, 1990.

Billings, Dwight B. "Religion as Opposition: A Gramscian Analysis." *American Journal of Sociology* 96, no. 1 (1990): 1–31.

Blaxton, Reginald Glenn. "'Jesus Wept': Reflects on HIV Dis-ease and the Churches of Black Folk." In *Dangerous Liaisons: Blacks, Gays, and the Struggle for Equality*, edited by Eric Brandt, 102–41. New York: The New Press, 1999.

Cadge, Wendy, and Lynn Davidman. "Ascription, Choice, and the Construction of Religious Identities in the Contemporary United States." *Journal for the Scientific Study of Religion* 45, no. 1 (2006): 23–38.

Centers for Disease Control and Prevention.HIV/AIDS Surveillance Report, 2004. Vol. 16. Atlanta, GA: U.S. Department of Health and Human Services, Centers for Disease Control and Prevention, 2005.

Centers for Disease Control and Prevention. "HIV among African Americans." Centers for Disease Control and Prevention, 2014a, accessed June 3, 2014. http://www.cdc.gov/hiv/risk/racialethnic/aa/facts/index.html.

Centers for Disease Control and Prevention. "Health Disparities in HIV/AIDS, Viral Hepatitis, STDs, and TB: African Americans/Blacks." Centers for Disease Control and Prevention, 2014b, accessed June 3, 2014. http://www.cdc.gov/nchhstp/healthdisparities/African-Americans.html.

Cohen, Cathy J. *Boundaries of Blackness: AIDS and the Breakdown of Black Politics.* Chicago: University of Chicago Press, 1999.

Collins, Patricia Hill. *Black Feminist Thought: Knowledge, Consciousness, and the Politics of Empowerment*, 2nd ed. New York: Routledge, 2000.

Collins, Patricia. *Black Sexual Politics: African Americans, Gender, and the New Racism*. New York: Routledge, 2004.

Cone, James H. *A Black Theology of Liberation*. Maryknoll, NY: Orbis Books, 1990.

Creswell, John W. *Research Design: Qualitative, Quantitative, and Mixed Methods Approaches*, 2nd ed. Thousand Oaks, CA: Sage Publications, 2003.

Doka, Kenneth J. *AIDS, Fear, and Society: Challenging the Dreaded Disease*. Bristol, PA: Taylor & Francis, 1997.

Douglas, Kelly Brown. *Sexuality and the Black Church: A Womanist Perspective*. Maryknoll, NY: Orbis Books, 1999.

Dufour, Lynn Resnick. "Sifting through Tradition: The creation of Jewish Feminist Identities." *Journal for the Scientific Study of Religion* 39, no. 1 (2000): 90–106.

Duneier, Mitchell. *Sidewalk*. New York: Farrar, Straus and Giroux, 1999.

Eliasoph, Nina, and Paul Lichterman. "Culture in Interaction." *American Journal of Sociology* 108, no. 4 (2003): 735–94.

Ellingson, Stephen, Nelson Tebbe, Martha van Haitsma, and Edward O. Laumann. "Religion and the Politics of Sexuality." *Journal of Contemporary Ethnography* 30, no. 1 (2001): 3–55.

Emerson, Robert M. *Contemporary Field Research: Perspectives and Formulations*, 2nd ed. Prospect Heights, IL: Waveland Press, Inc., 2001.

Fine, Gary A. "Ten Lies of Ethnography: Moral Dilemmas in Field Research." *Journal of Contemporary Ethnography* 22 (1993): 267–94.

Frederick, Marla F. *Between Sundays: Black Women and Everyday Struggles of Faith*. Berkeley, CA: University of California Press, 2003.

Freimuth, Vicki S., Sandra Crouse Quinn, Stephen B. Thomas, Galen Cole, Eric Zook, and Ted Duncan. "African Americans' Views on Research and the Tuskegee Syphilis Study." *Social Science & Medicine* 52, no. 5 (2001): 797–808.

Freudenberg, Nick. "Health Promotion in the City: A Review of Current Practice and Future Prospects in the United States." *Annual Review of Public Health* 21 (2000): 473–503.

Gilkes, Cheryl Townsend. "The Roles of Church and Community Mothers: Ambivalent American Sexism or Fragmented African Familyhood." *Journal of Feminist Studies in Religion* 2, no. 1 (1986): 41–59.

Glaser, Barney G., and Anselm L. Strauss. *The Discovery of Grounded Theory: Strategies for Qualitative Research*. New York: Aldine de Gruyter, 1967.

Greer, Bruce A., and Wade Clark Roof. "'Desperately Seeking Sheila': Locating Religious Privatism in American Society." *Journal for the Scientific Study of Religion* 31, no. 3 (1992): 346–52.

Gutierrez, Gustavo. *A Theology of Liberation*. Maryknoll, NY: Orbis Books, 1973.

Hammonds, Evelynn M. "Seeing AIDS: Race, Gender, and Representation." In *The Gender Politics of HIV/AIDS in Women*, edited by Nancy Goldstein and Jennifer Manlowe, 113–126. New York: New York University Press, 1997.

Hunter, James Davison. *American Evangelicalism*. New Brunswick, NJ: Rutgers University Press, 1983.

Idler, Ellen L. "Religious Involvement and the Health of the Elderly: Some Hypotheses and an Initial Test." *Social Forces* 66, no. 1 (1987): 226–38.

Jacobson, Jr., C. Jeff, Sara E. Luckhaupt, Sheli Delaney, and Joel Tsevat. "Religio-Biography, Coping, and Meaning-Making among Persons with HIV/AIDS." *Journal for the Scientific Study of Religion* 45, no. 1 (2006): 39–56.

Krouse, Mary Beth. "Feminist Discursive Pivoting: Charting the Politics of AIDS." *Humanity & Society* 23, no. 1 (1999): 32–48.

Lasch, Christopher. *The Culture of Narcissism: American Life in an Age of Diminishing Expectations*. New York: W.W. Norton & Company, 1979.

Leong, Pamela. "Religion, Flesh, and Blood: Re-creating Religious Culture in the Context of HIV/AIDS." *Sociology of Religion* 67, no. 3 (2006): 295–311.

Lichterman, Paul. *The Search for Political Community: American Activists Reinventing Commitment.* New York: Cambridge University Press, 1996.

Lincoln, C. Eric, and Lawrence H. Mamiya. *The Black Church in the African American Experience.* Durham, NC: Duke University Press, 1990.

Lorde, Audre. "Age, Race, Class and Sex: Women Redefining Difference." In *Gender Through the Prism of Difference*, 2nd ed., edited by Maxine Baca Zinn, Pierrette Hondagneu-Sotelo, and Michael A. Messner, 503–508. Reprint, Needham Heights, MA: Allyn & Bacon, [1984] 2000.

May, Gerald G. *Addiction and Grace.* New York: Harper & Row, 1988.

Mays, Benjamin, and Joseph Nicholson. *The Negro's Church.* Reprint, New York: Russell and Russell, [1933] 1969.

McGuire, Meredith B. "Why Bodies Matter: A Sociological Reflection on Spirituality and Materiality," *Spiritus* 3, no.1 (2003): 1–18.

McRoberts, Omar M. *Streets of Glory: Church and Community in a Black Urban Neighborhood.* Chicago: University of Chicago Press, 2003.

Miceli, Melinda S. "Morality Politics vs. Identity Politics: Framing Processes and Competition among Christian Right and Gay Social Movement Organizations." *Sociological Forum* 20, no. 4 (2005): 589–612.

Mitchell, Claire. "Behind the Ethnic Marker: Religion and Social Identification in Northern Ireland." *Sociology of Religion* 66, no. 1 (2005): 3–21.

Moon, Dawne. *God, Sex, and Politics: Homosexuality and Everyday Theologies.* Chicago: University of Chicago Press, 2004.

Morris, Aldon D. *The Origins of the Civil Rights Movement: Black Communities Organizing for Change.* New York: Free Press, 1984.

Muhr, Thomas. *User's Manual for ATLAS.ti 5.0,* ATLAS.ti Scientific Software Development GmbH, Berlin, 2004.

Myrdal, Gunnar. *An American Dilemma: The Negro Problem and Modern Democracy.* Reprint, New Brunswick, NJ: Transaction Publishers, [1944] 1996.

Office of Minority Health, U.S. Department of Health and Human Services. "HIV/AIDS and African Americans." Office of Minority Health, U.S. Department of Health and Human Services. 2013. Accessed June 3, 2014. http://minorityhealth.hhs.gov/templates/content.aspx?ID=3019.

Oswald, Ramona Faith. "Resilience within the Family Networks of Lesbians and Gay Men: Intentionality and Redefinition." *Journal of Marriage and Family* 64, no. 2 (2002): 374–83.

Pharr, Suzanne. *Homophobia: A Weapon of Sexism.* Berkeley, CA: Chardon Press, 1997.

Pilla, Anthony M. "A Healing Presence." *Health Progress* (May–June 2001): 15–20.

Pinn, Anthony B. "Black Bodies in Pain and Ecstasy: Terror, Subjectivity, and the Nature of Black Religion." *Nova Religio: The Journal of Alternative and Emergent Religions* 7, no. 1 (2003): 76–89.

Pope, Stephen. "Expressive Individualism and True Self-Love: A Thomistic Perspective." *The Journal of Religion* 71, no. 3 (1991): 384–99.

Putnam, Robert D. *Bowling Alone: The Collapse and Revival of American Community.* New York: Simon & Schuster, 2000.

Read, Jen'Nan Ghazal, and John P. Bartkowski. "To Veil or Not to Veil? A Case Study of Identity Negotiation among Muslim Women in Austin, Texas." *Gender and Society* 14, no. 3 (2000): 395–417.

Rich, Adrienne. "Compulsory Heterosexuality and Lesbian Existence." *Signs* 5, no. 4 (1980): 631–60.

Rieff, Philip. *The Triumph of the Therapeutic: Uses of Faith After Freud.* Reprint, Chicago: University of Chicago Press, [1966] 1987.

Rieff, Philip. *Freud: The Mind of the Moralist..* Garden City, NY: Anchor Books, 1961.

Rodriguez, Eric M., and Suzanne C. Ouellette. "Gay and Lesbian Christians: Homosexual and Religious Identity Integration in the Members and Participants of a Gay-Positive Church." *Journal for the Scientific Study of Religion* 39, no. 3 (2000): 333–47.

Roof, Wade Clark. *Spiritual Marketplace: Baby Boomers and the Remaking of American Religion.* Princeton, NJ: Princeton University Press, 1999.

Sargeant, Kimon Howland. *Seeker Churches: Promoting Traditional Religion in Nontradition-al Ways.* New Brunswick, NJ: Rutgers University Press, 2000.

Schieman, Scott, Tetyana Pudrovska, Leonard I. Pearlin, and Christopher G. Ellison. "The Sense of Divine Control and Psychological Distress: Variations Across Race and Socioeconomic Status." *Journal for the Scientific Study of Religion* 45, no. 4 (2006): 529–49.

Schlesinger, Jr., Arthur M. *The Disuniting of America.* New York: W.W. Norton, 1992.

Shallenberger, David. *Reclaiming the Spirit: Gay Men and Women Come to Terms with Religion.* New Brunswick, NJ: Rutgers University Press, 1998.

Smith, Christian. *The Emergence of Liberation Theology: Radical Religion and Social Movement Theory.* Chicago: University of Chicago Press, 1991.

Stine, Gerald J. *AIDS Update 1999.* Upper Saddle River, NJ: Prentice Hall, 1999.

Strauss, Anselm, and Juliet Corbin. *Basics of Qualitative Research: Grounded Theory Procedures and Techniques.* Newbury Park, CA: Sage Publications, 1990.

Swidler, Ann. *Talk of Love: How Culture Matters.* Chicago: University of Chicago Press, 2001.

Swidler, Ann. "Culture in Action: Symbols and Strategies." *American Sociological Review* 51, no. 2 (1986): 273–86.

Thomson, Irene Taviss. "The Theory That Won't Die: From Mass Society to the Decline of Social Capital." *Sociological Forum* 20, no. 3 (2005): 421–48.

Thorne, Barrie. "'You Still Takin' Notes?' Fieldwork and Problems of Informed Consent." *Social Problems* 27, no. 3 (1980): 284–97.

Thurman, Howard. "The Anatomy of Segregation and Ground of Hope." In *African American Religious History: A Documentary Witness,* 2nd ed., edited by Milton C. Sernett, 548–54. Reprint, Durham, NC: Duke University Press, [1965] 1999.

Tocqueville, Alexis de. *Democracy in America.* Edited and abridged by Richard D. Heffner. New York: Signet Classic, 2001.

Unity Fellowship Church. "Unity Fellowship Church: History." Unity Fellowship Church of Christ Church, Inc. Accessed January 31, 2007. http:// http://www.ufc-usa.org/history.html.

United States Census Bureau. "State and County QuickFacts." United States Census Bureau. Accessed June 2, 2014. http://quickfacts.census.gov/qfd/states/00000.html.

Walker, Wyatt Tee. "The Contemporary Black Church." In *The Black Church: A Community Resource,* edited by Dionne J. Jones and William H. Matthews, 36–68. Reprint, Washington, DC.: Institute for Urban Affairs and Research, Howard University, [1976] 1977.

Weatherford, Ronald Jeffrey, and Carole Boston Weatherford. *Somebody's Knocking at Your Door: AIDS and the African-American Church.* Binghamton, NY: Haworth Press, Inc., 1998.

Wilcox, Melissa M. "When Sheila's a Lesbian: Religious Individualism among Lesbian, Gay, Bisexual, and Transgender Christians." *Sociology of Religion* 63, no. 4 (2002): 497–513.

Wilcox, Melissa M. "Of Markets and Missions: The Early History of the Universal Fellowship of Metropolitan Community Churches." *Religion and American Culture: A Journal of Interpretation* 11, no. 1 (2001): 83–108.

Williams, Rhys H. "Constructing the Public Good: Social Movements and Cultural Resources." *Social Problems* 42, no. 1 (1995): 124–44.

Wilson, Bryan. *Religion in Sociological Perspective.* Oxford: Oxford University Press, 1982.

Wolkomir, Michelle. "Wrestling with the Angels of Meaning: The Revisionist Ideological Work of Gay and Ex-Gay Christian Men." *Symbolic Interaction* 24, no. 4 (2001): 407–24.

Wuthnow, Robert. *After Heaven: Spirituality in America Since the 1950s.* Berkeley, CA: University of California Press, 1998.

Wuthnow, Robert, ed. *Vocabularies of Public Life: Empirical Essays in Symbolic Structure.* New York: Routledge, 1992.

Yamane, David. "A Sociologist Comments on Sommerville: The Whole Is Less Than the Sum of its Part." *Journal for the Scientific Study of Religion* 37, no. 2 (1998): 254–56.

Yamane, David. "Secularization on Trial: In Defense of a Neo-Secularization Paradigm." *Journal for the Scientific Study of Religion* 36, no. 1 (1997): 109–22.

Yip, Andrew K. T. "The Persistence of Faith among Nonheterosexual Christians: Evidence for the Neosecularization Thesis of Religious Transformation." *Journal for the Scientific Study of Religion* 41, no. 2 (2002): 199–212.

Index

AIDS. *See* HIV/AIDS
anomy, 7, 39, 40
Archbishop Carl Bean. *See* Bean, Carl

Bean, Carl, 19–23, 126; AIDS crisis,
    response to, 19, 34; background, 19–23,
    28; communication style and language,
    29, 80–82; entertainer, 35; high profile,
    12; Minority AIDS Project, founding,
    19; permissiveness, 97–98; religious
    influences, 20, 28; religious trajectory,
    20, 36n5, 36n8; social justice, 21;
    symbolism, 127; theology, 22, 29;
    therapist, 31, 34, 82, 123, 127; Unity
    Fellowship Church, founding, 19
Bellah, Robert et al., *Habits of the Heart*,
    10
Bible: contradictions, 59; GLBT issues, 59.
    See also personalized religion,
    individual strategies, sifting;
    personalized religion, bible,
    recognizing as man-made
black churches, 15n7, 27; autonomy, 6;
    congregational practices, 22, 27, 28;
    embodied practices, 28, 33;
    homophobic, 1, 4; importance of, 6–7;
    mystification of, 7–8, 8; response to
    HIV/AIDS, 3–6; social justice, 6–7

churches. *See also* black churches ;
    congregational compatibility: gay-
    affirming churches, 27, 48–49, 51;
    homophobia, 23–24, 25, 40, 43, 85;
    traditional churches, 34, 42, 44, 85
Collins, Patricia Hill, 105–106, 110
congregational compatibility, 27;
    Afrocentric, 27, 51–52; affirmation of
    GLBT status, 27, 42, 44, 49; church
    hopping/shopping, 25–26, 26, 39, 44,
    115; freeing, 43, 45; need to be
    spiritually fed, 47–48; non-oppressive,
    45; open and honest dialogue from the
    pulpit, 49; sense of belonging, comfort,
    and fit, 44, 45, 46; traditional religious
    traditions, 49–51, 52, 72
culture. *See also* remissive cultures. *See
    also* Unity Fellowship church, cultural
    practices

Dufour, Lynn Resnick, 60

Freud, Sigmund, 31, 82, 97, 127

gay churches. *See* churches, gay-affirming
    churches; Metropolitan Community
    Church; Unity Fellowship Church
gay, lesbian, bisexual and/or transgender.
    See GLBT
gender: gender and the black church, 108,
    110–111; sexism and homophobia,
    107–110

155

About the Author

Pamela Leong is an assistant professor of sociology at Salem State University in Salem, Massachusetts.

CPSIA information can be obtained at www.ICGtesting.com
Printed in the USA
BVOW07*1247280415

397683BV00004B/5/P